Getting Ready My Adenoid Surgery

Adenoids Book for Kids – Preparation and Recovery

This book belongs to:

_____

Written by Dr. Fei Zheng-Ward   Illustrated by Moch. Fajar Shobaru

Copyright © 2024 Fei Zheng-Ward

All rights reserved. Published by Fei Zheng-Ward, an imprint of FZWbooks. No part of this book may be copied, reproduced, recorded, transmitted, or stored by any means or in any form, electronic or mechanical, without obtaining prior written permission from the copyright owner.

Identifiers: ISBN 979-8-89318-028-2 (eBook)
ISBN 979-8-89318-029-9 (paperback)
ISBN 979-8-89318-068-8 (hardcover)

What are adenoids?

They are one of many parts of your immune system that trap and fight germs to keep you healthy and strong.

Your adenoids are very hard to see because they hide out of sight in the back of your nose.

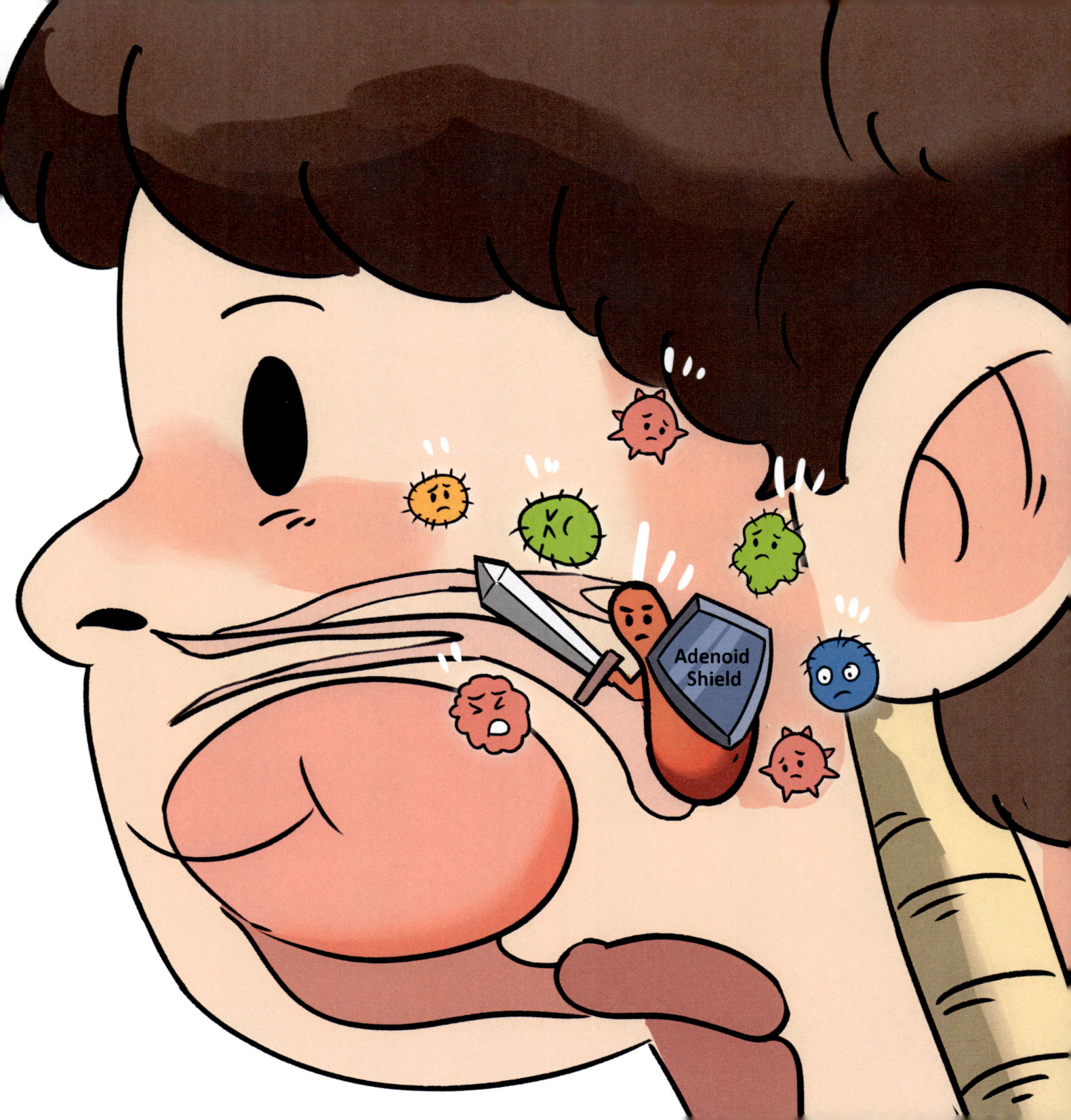

Your adenoids can get sick, too.

When that happens, they get
red and **swollen**.

Usually, they get better on their own.

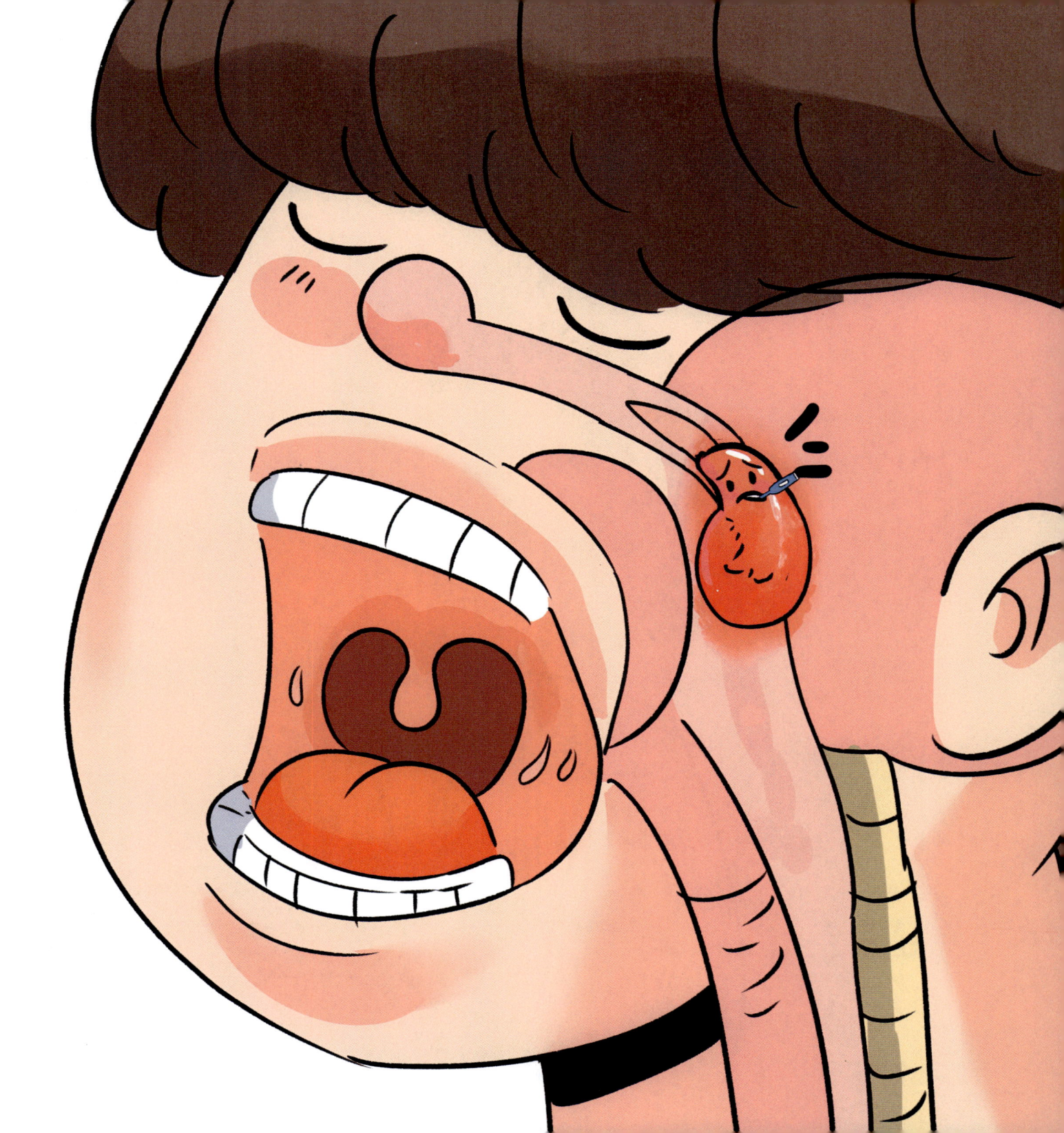

When they don't, your doctor may give you some medicine to take to help them get better.

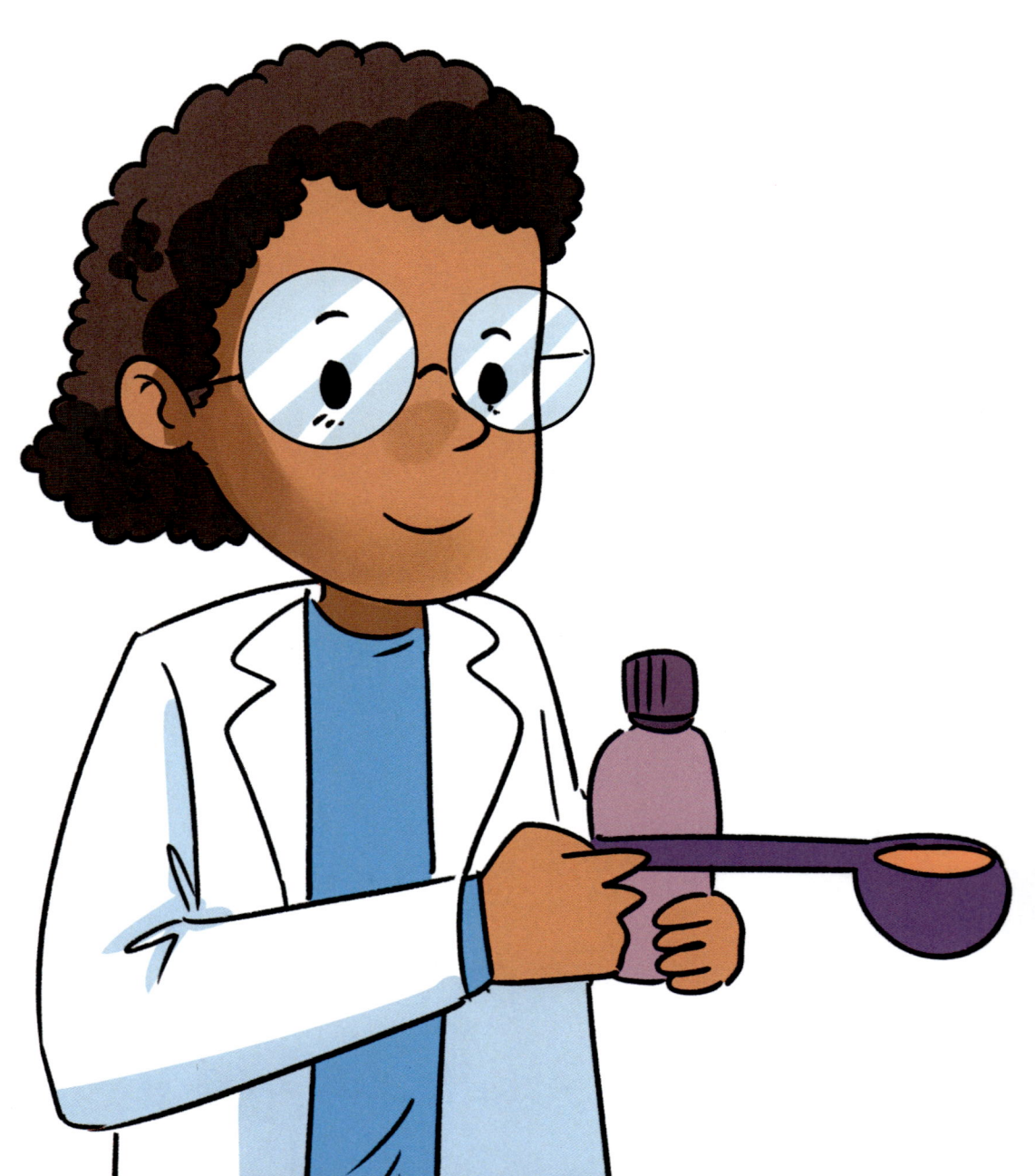

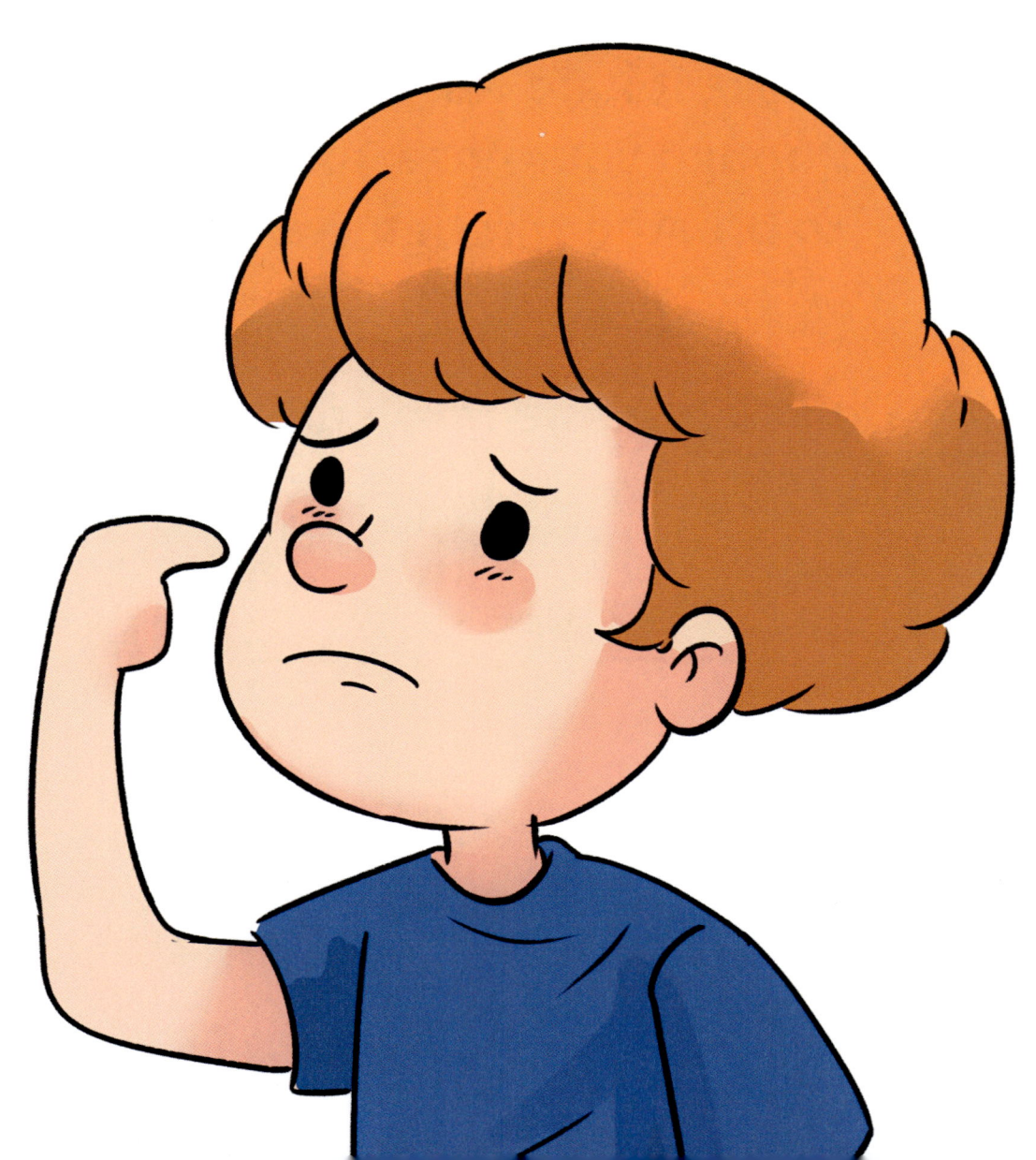

Sometimes, your adenoids can make it hard for you to breathe through your nose, and you have to breathe through your mouth.

Do you breathe through your mouth?

_____ YES   _____ NO

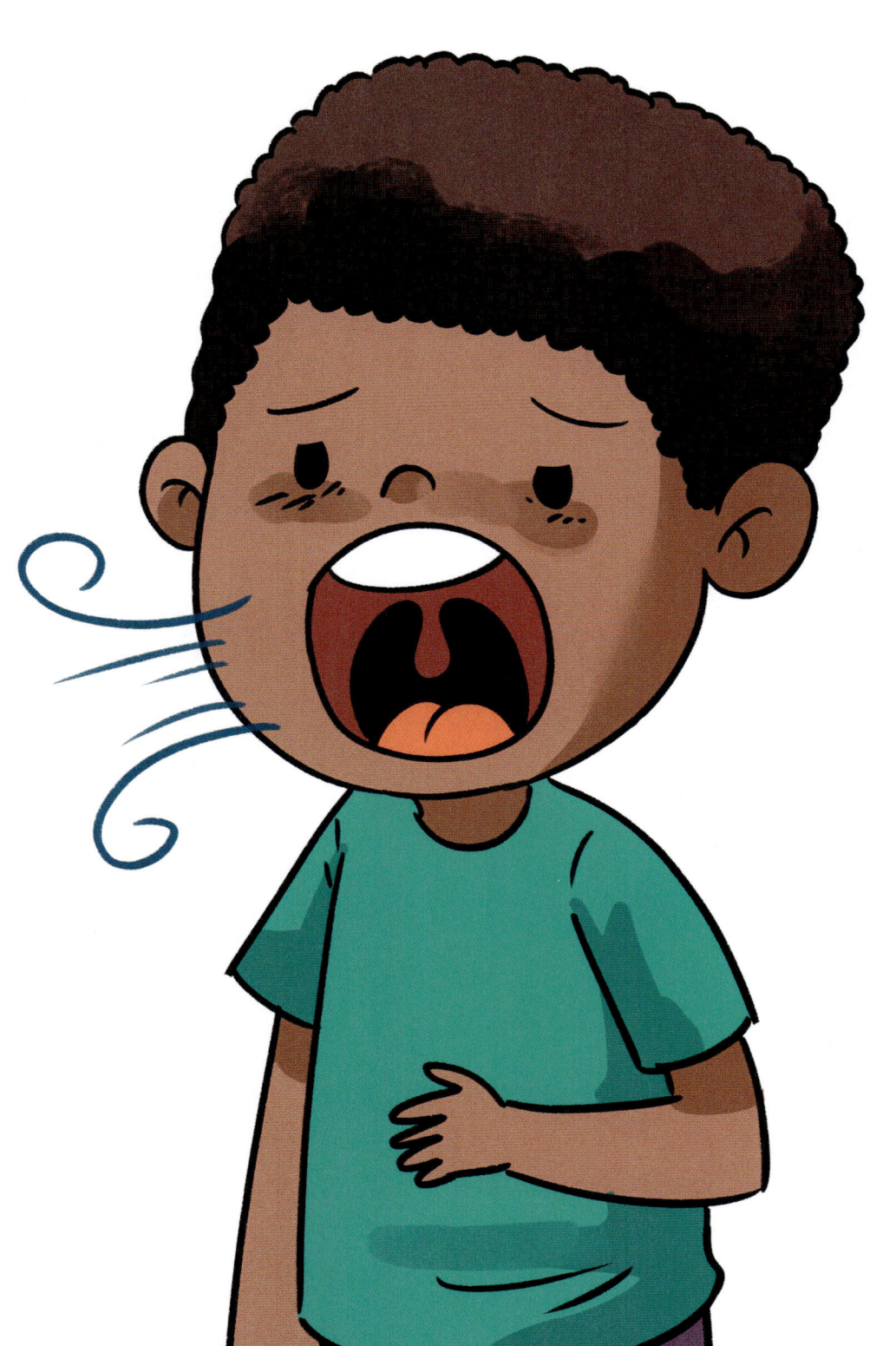

Or your stuffy nose may make silly musical sounds when you breathe.

Have you heard your nose make funny noises?

_____ YES   _____ NO

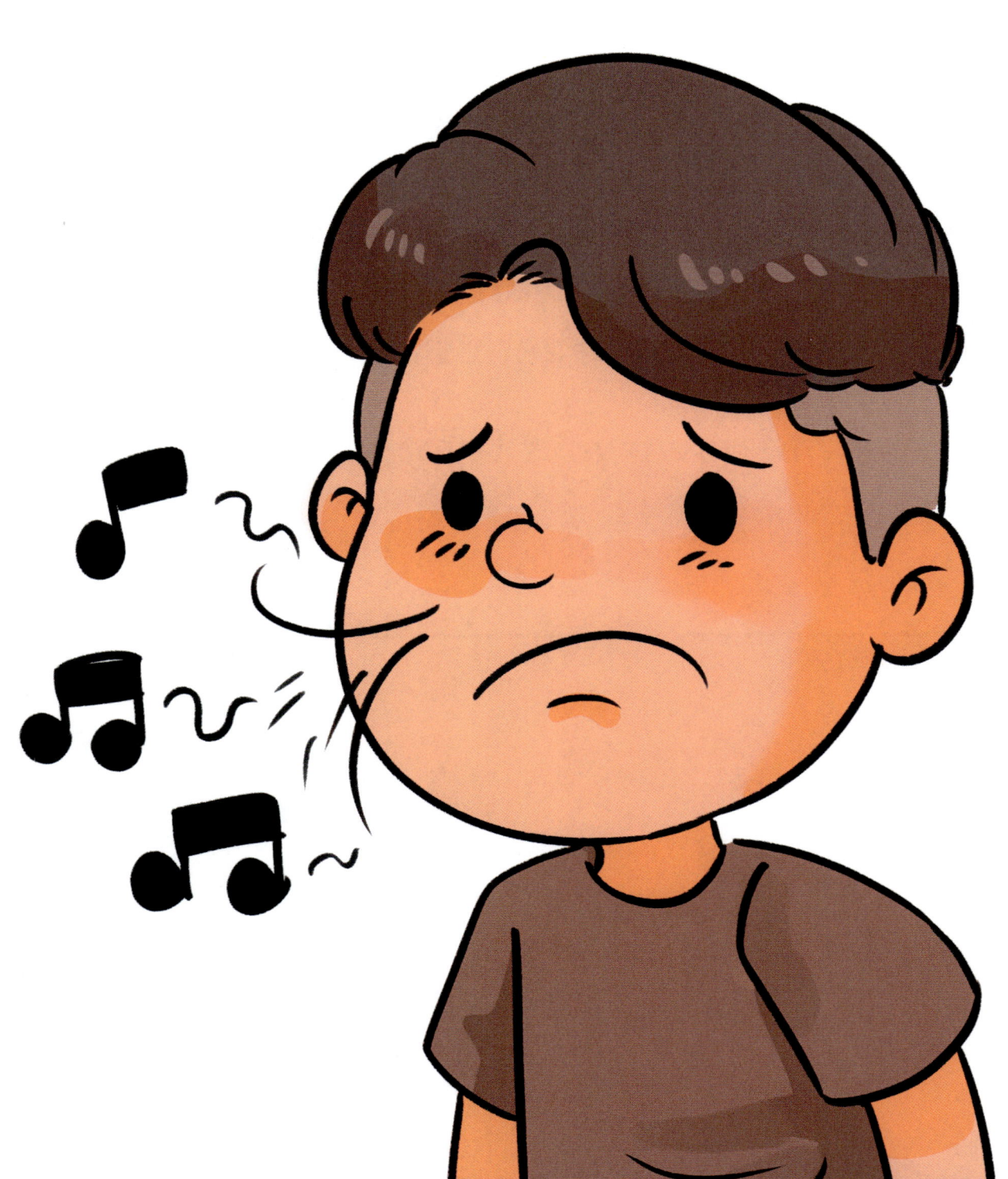

It can be hard to breathe
when your nose feels stuffy.

But try to drink water, some juice, or your favorite drink to stay hydrated so you can help your body fight the germs and get better.

Please write down your favorite drink below.

_____

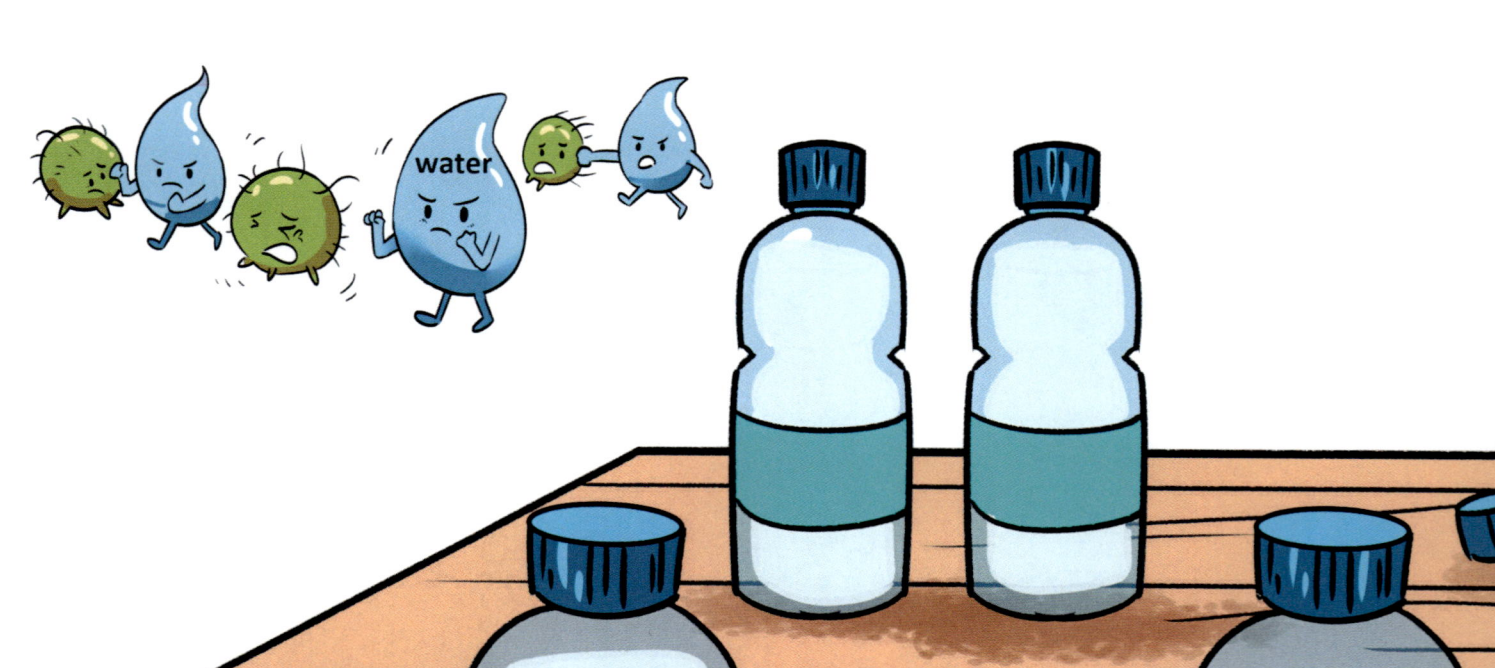

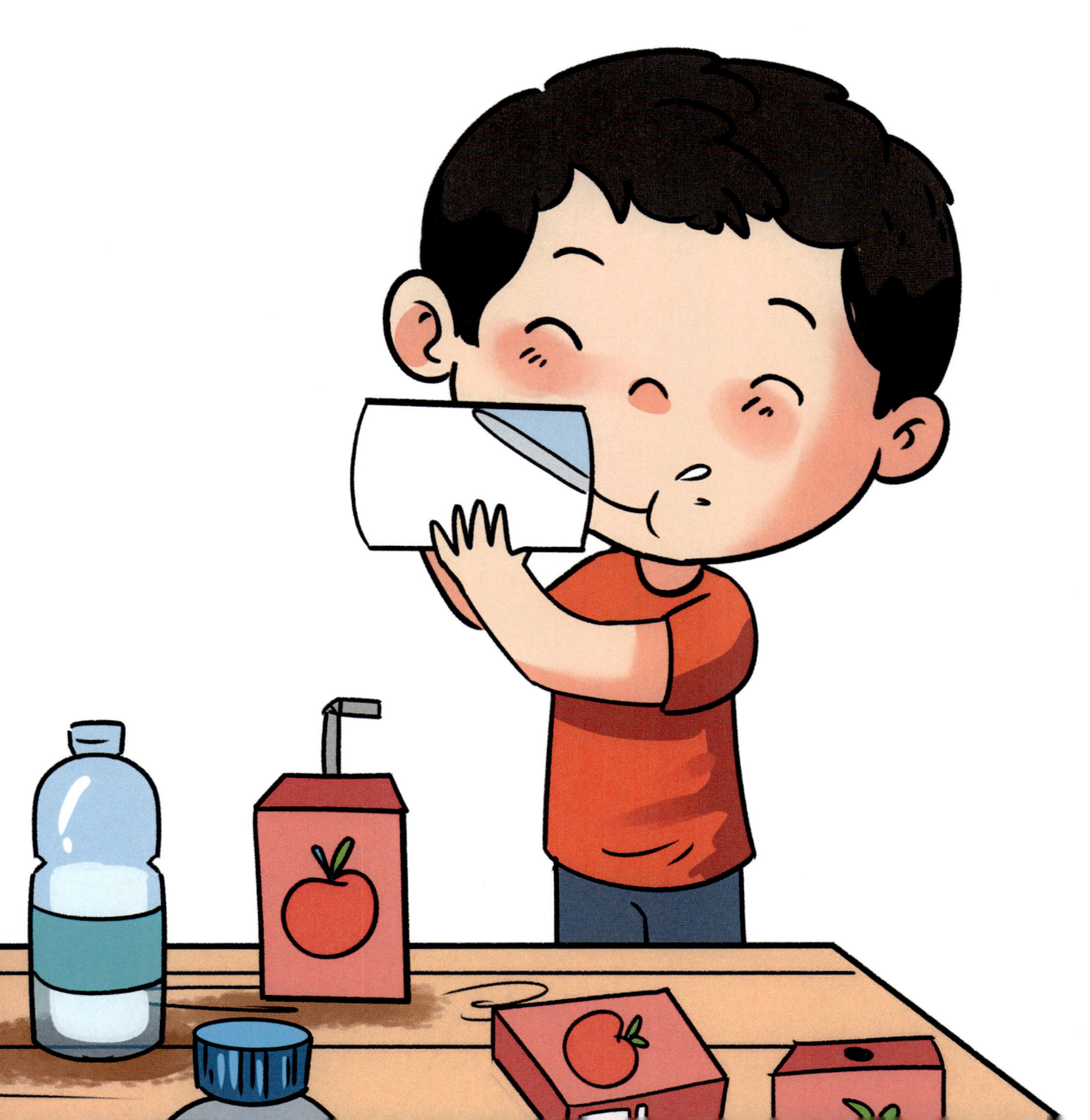

Your swollen adenoids may make you snore loudly like a bear.

Did anyone tell you you snore at night?

____ YES   ____ NO

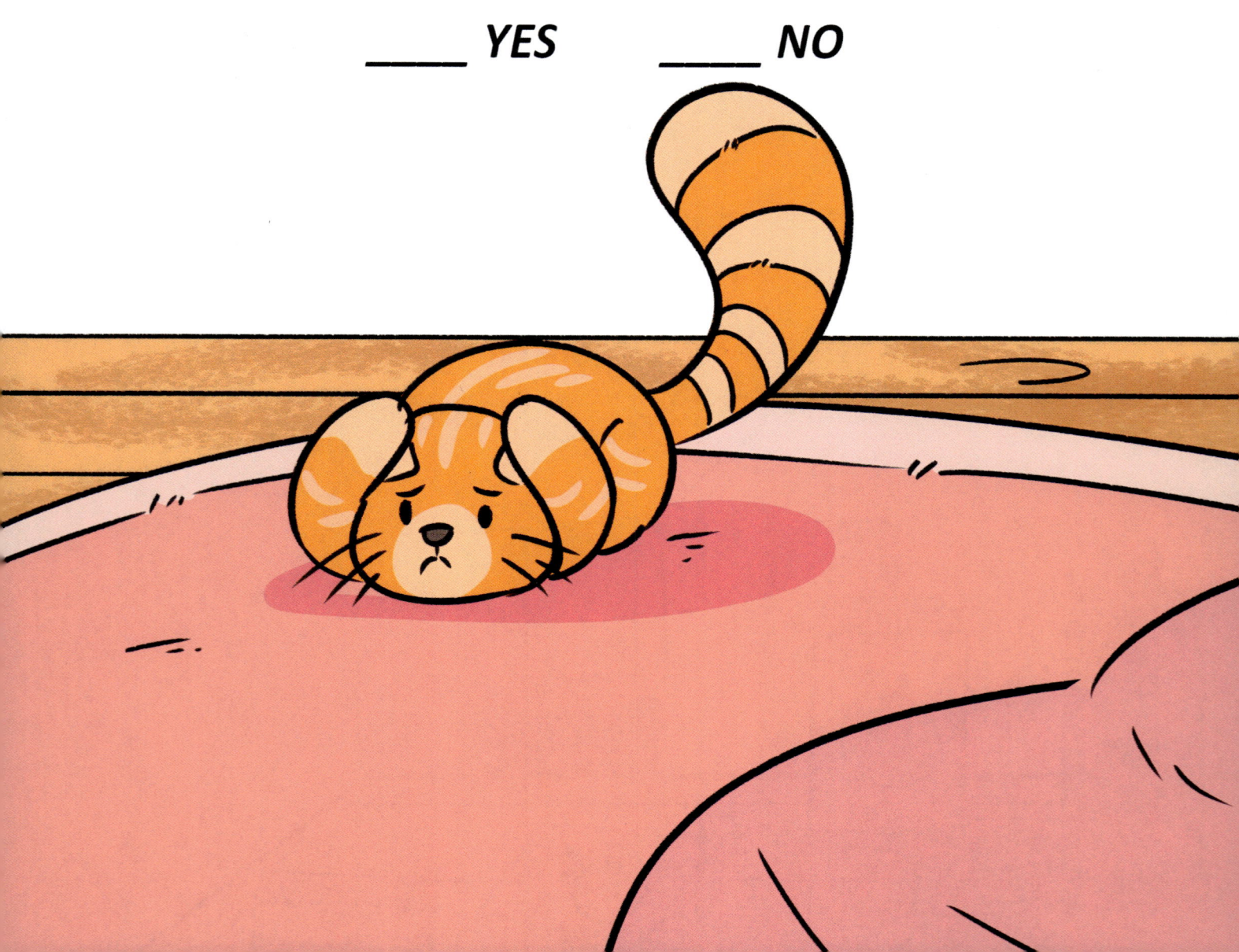

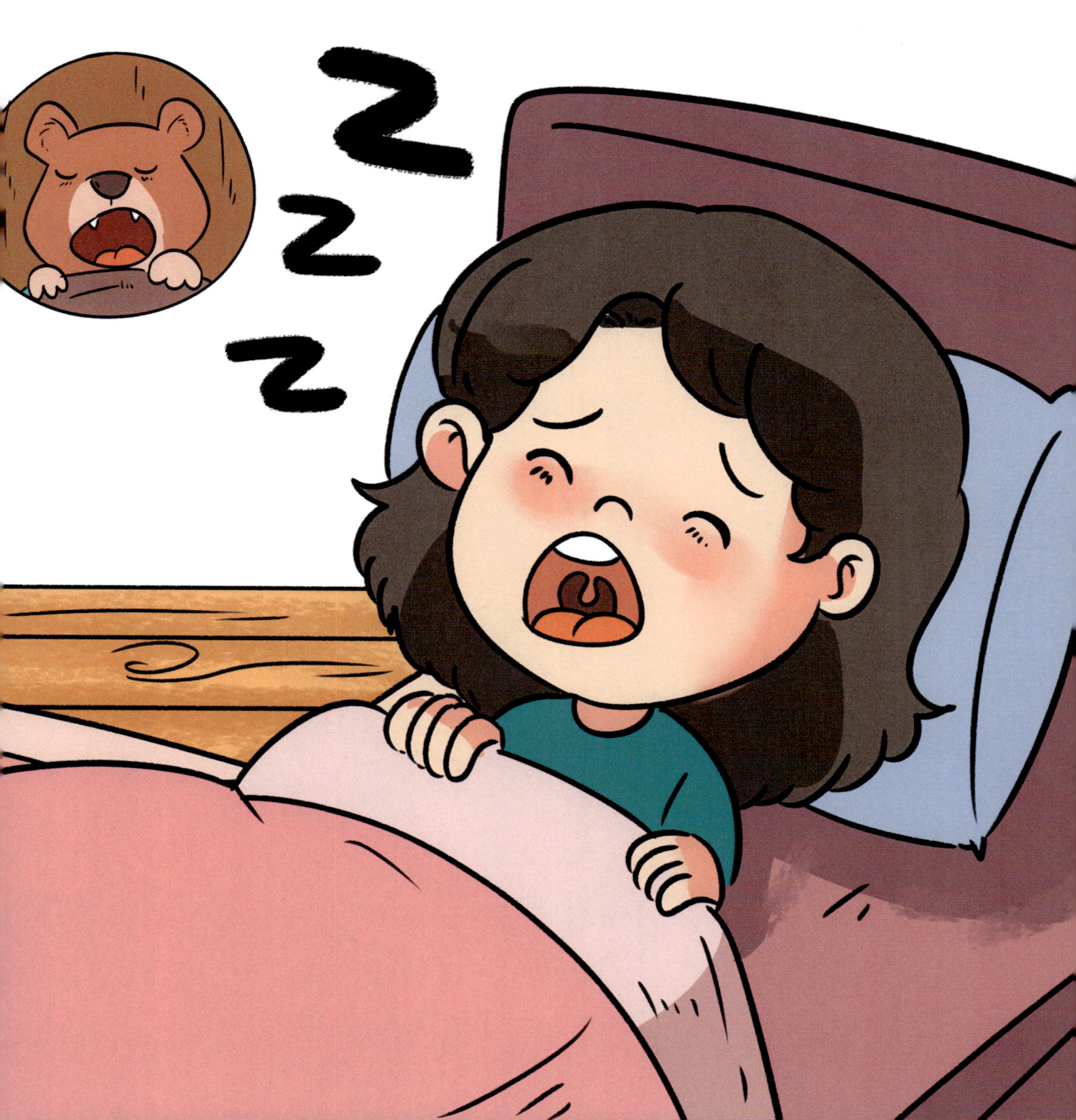

Sometimes, your adenoids keep getting sick, which can make you sick as well.

You may have a fever, sore throat, headache, earache, stuffy and runny nose, stinky breath, and don't want to eat much.

Has any of that happened to you?

____ YES   ____ NO

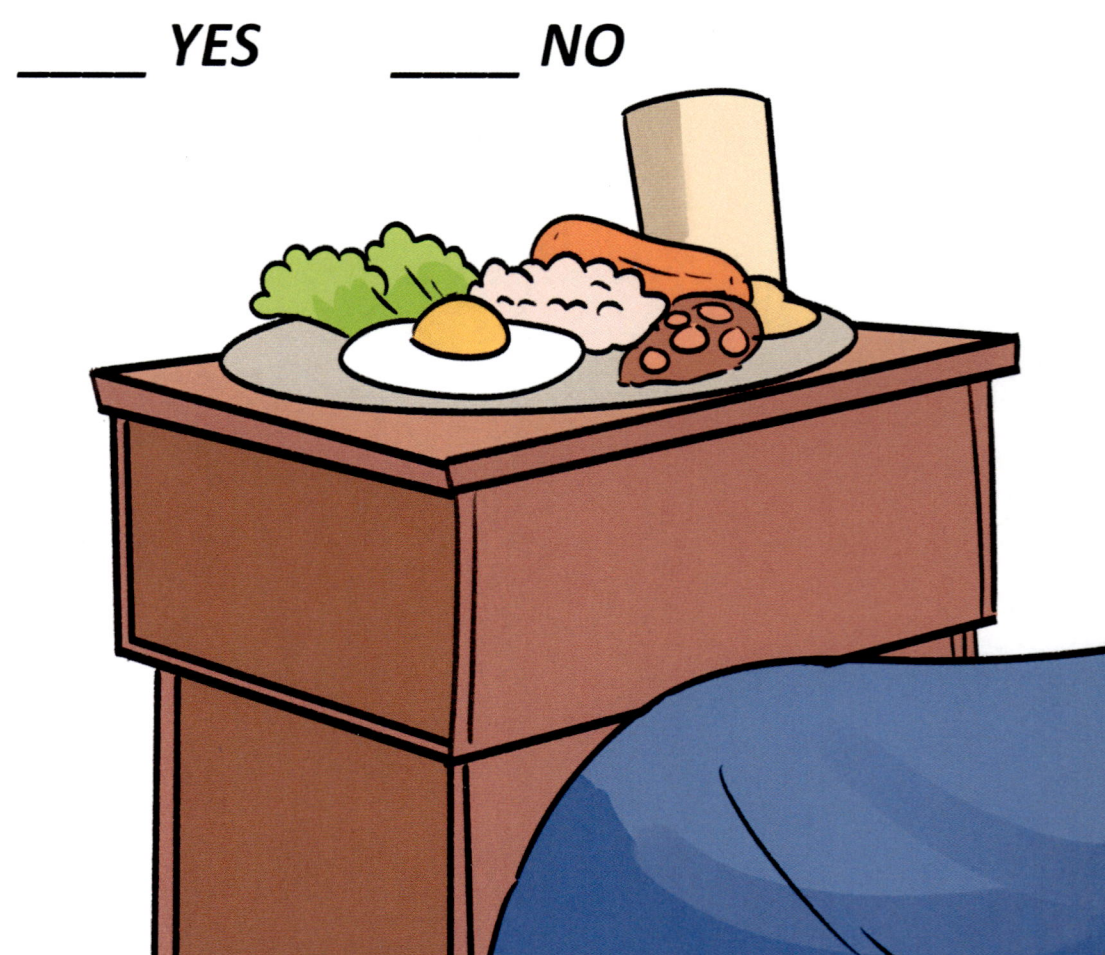

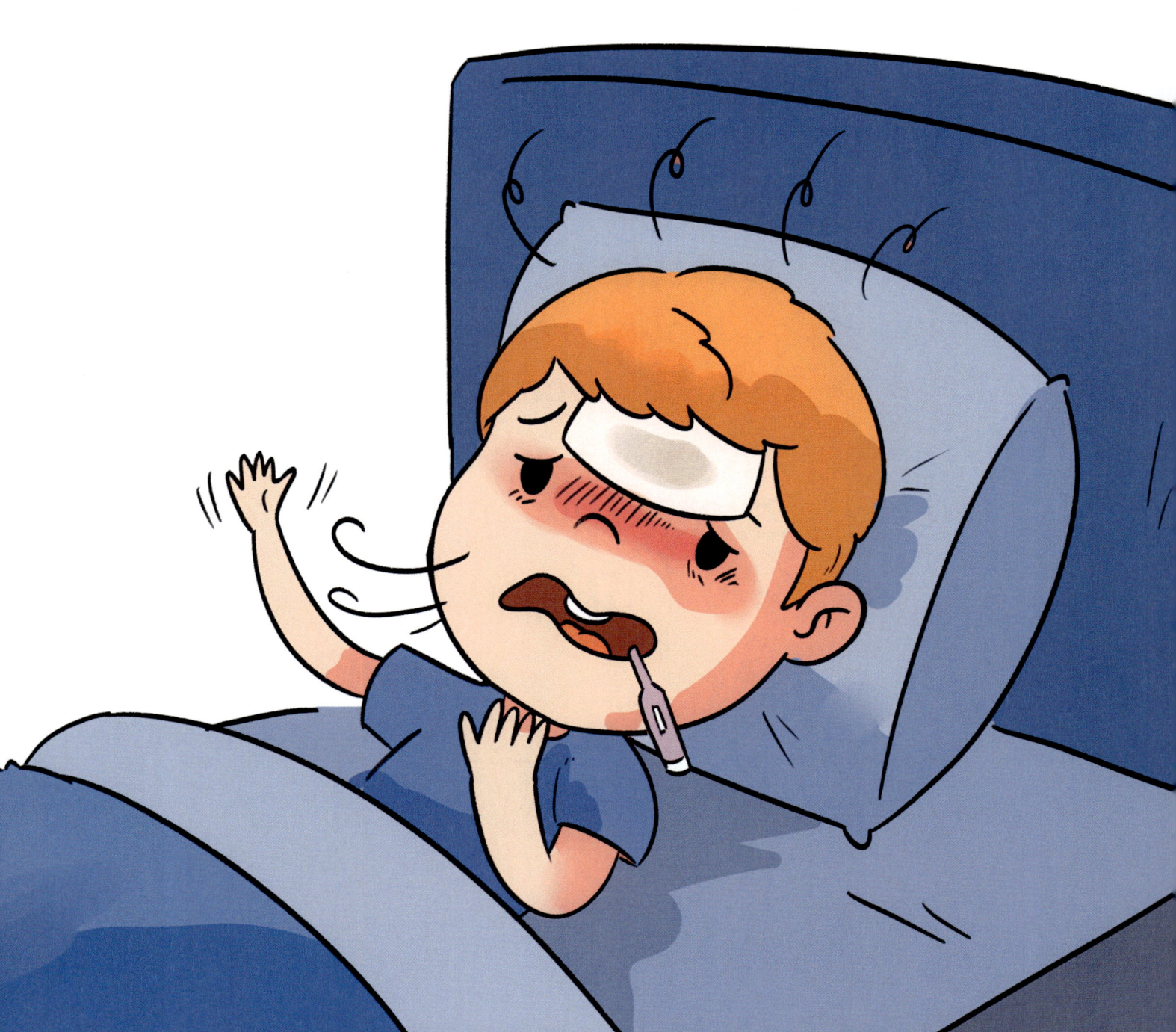

Your doctor, who is caring and gentle, can listen to your heart and lungs and check your ears, nose, and mouth.

Sometimes, they may recommend to have your adenoids removed so you can feel better.

Did your doctor say your adenoids are
big?

____ YES   ____ NO

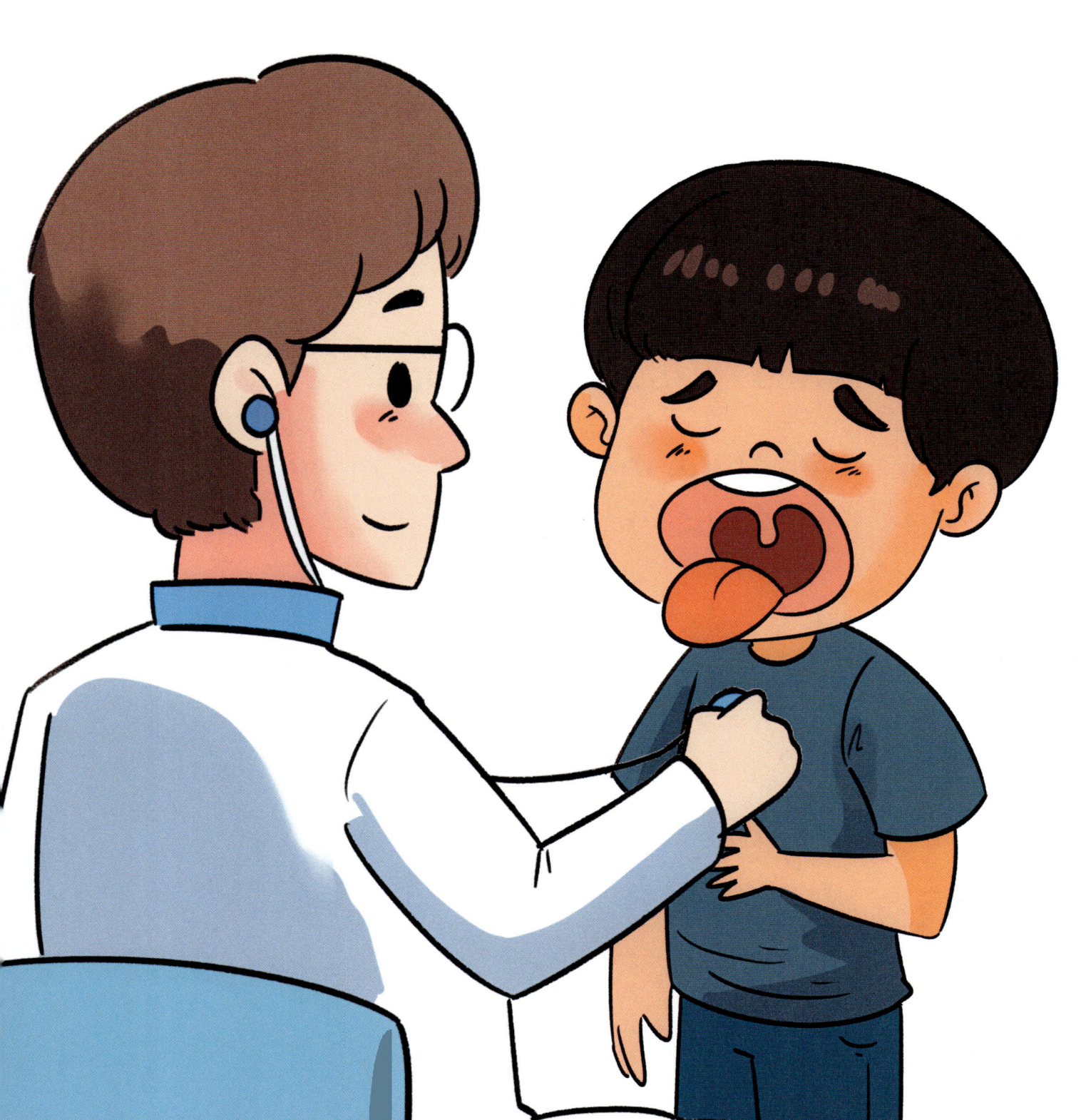

Your doctor can easily remove your
adenoids through your mouth.
It is a quick and simple surgery,
and you won't feel a thing!

You will be sleeping and dreaming away
while the surgery is underway.

*What do you want to dream
about for your surgery?*

Your adenoids will be all gone before you
wake up from your surgery.

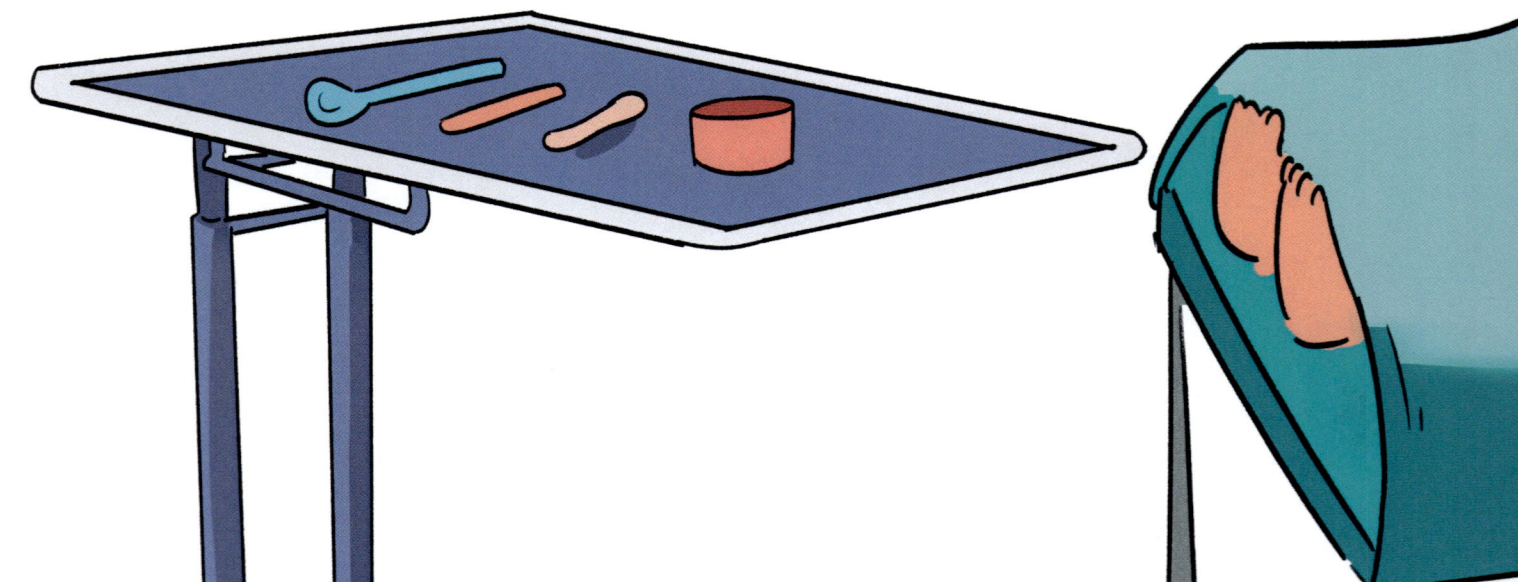

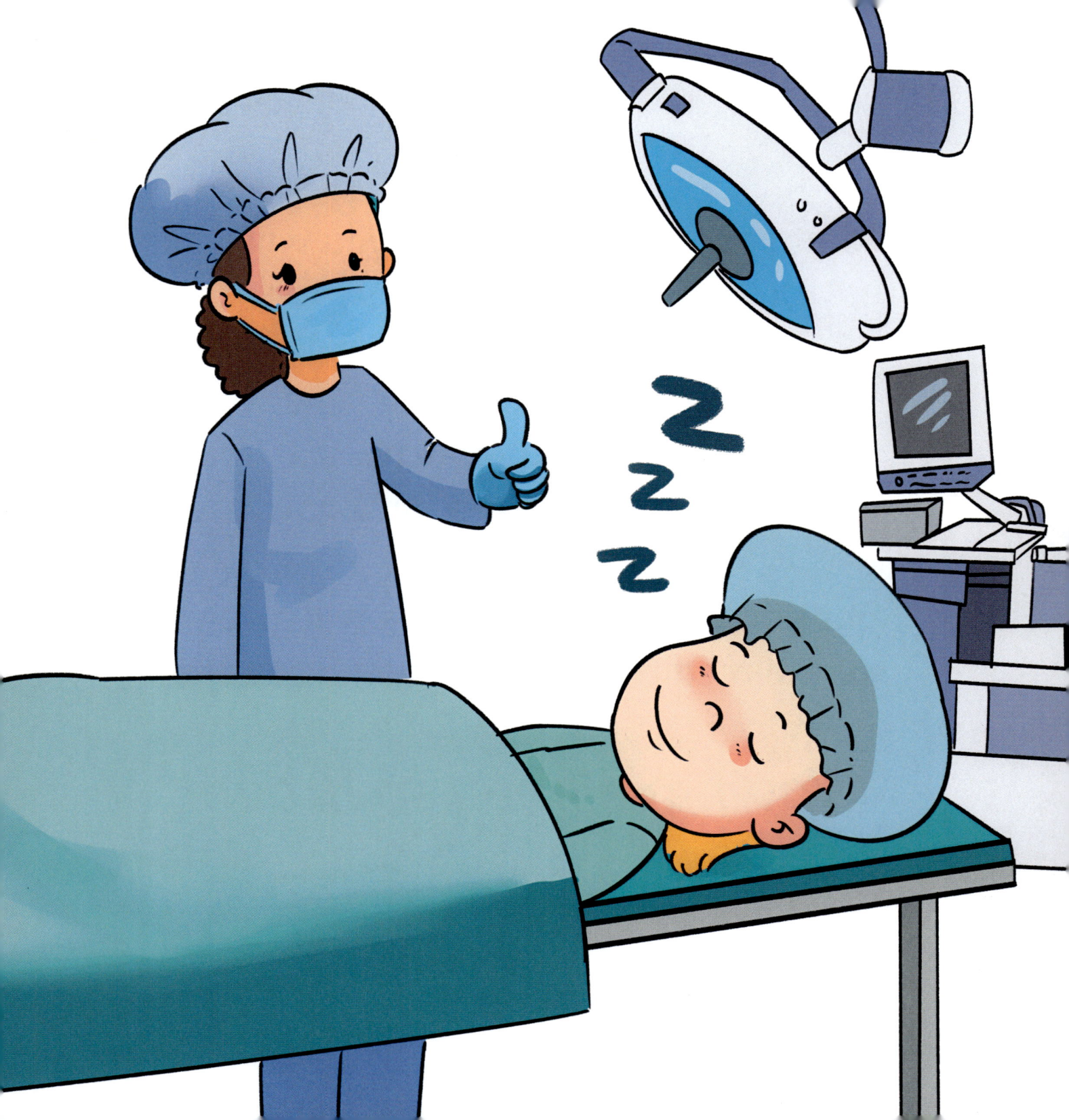

After your surgery is done, you will wake up in the hospital recovery room.

You may feel uncomfortable, your throat may feel sore and scratchy, and your breathing may be a little noisy.

But don't worry, your nurse will give you special medicine to make you feel better.

You have been so brave!

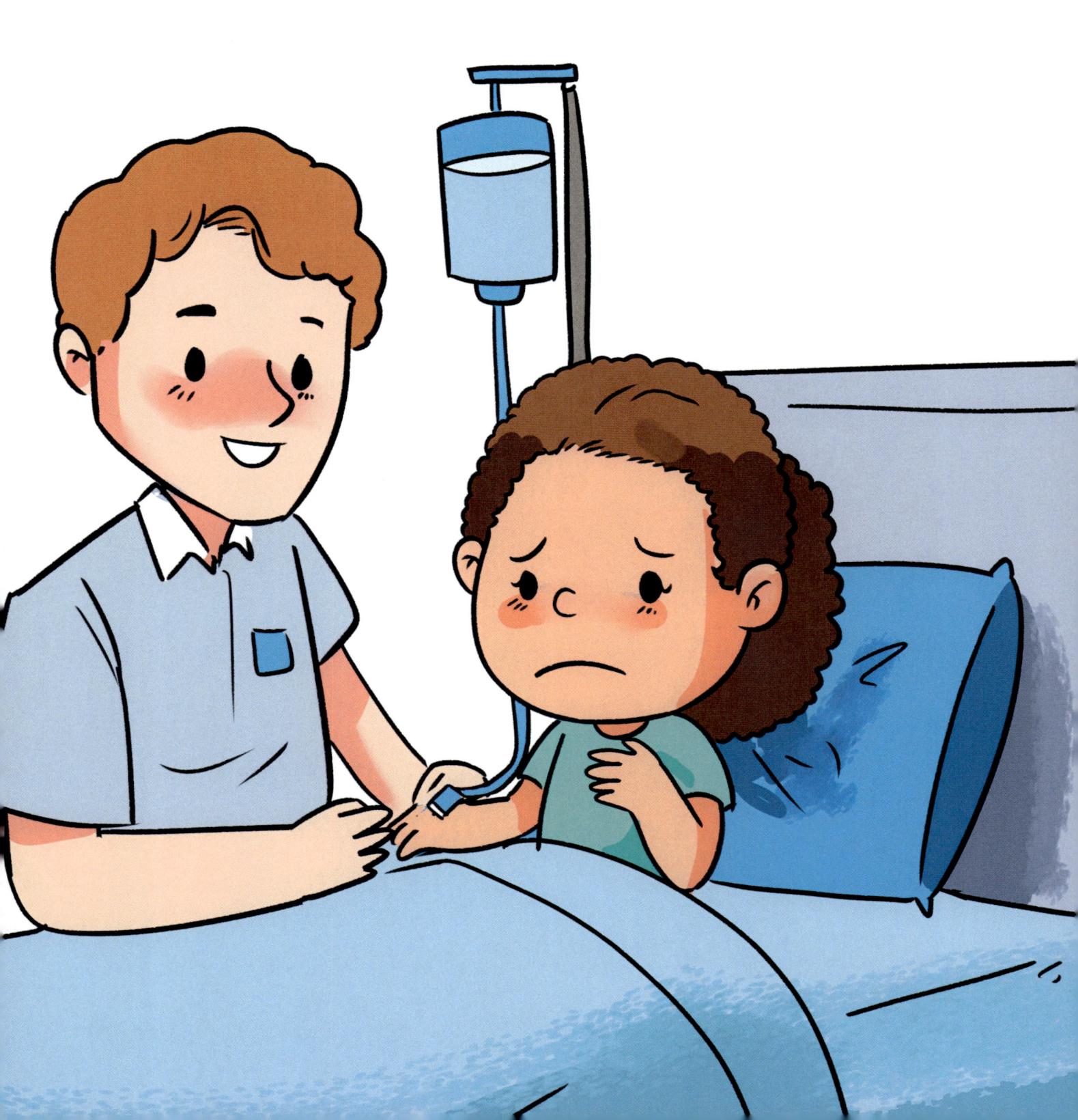

Sometimes, you may have to stay in the hospital after your surgery.

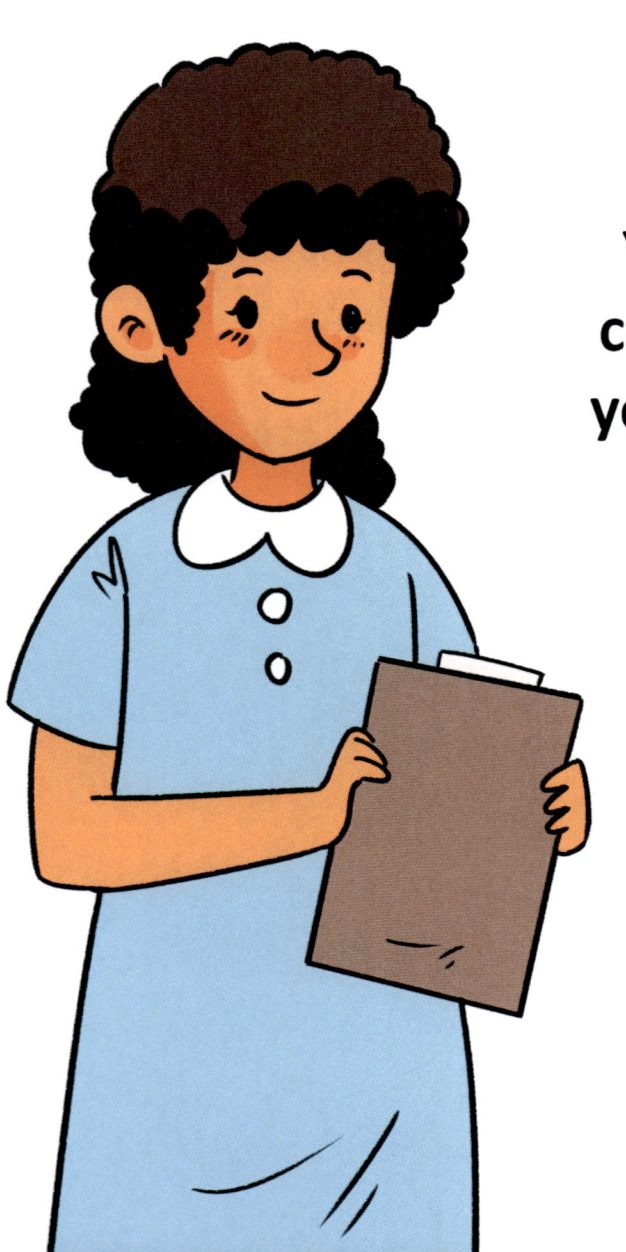

Your parent or guardian can stay with you to keep you safe and comfortable.

You can go home once you're feeling better.

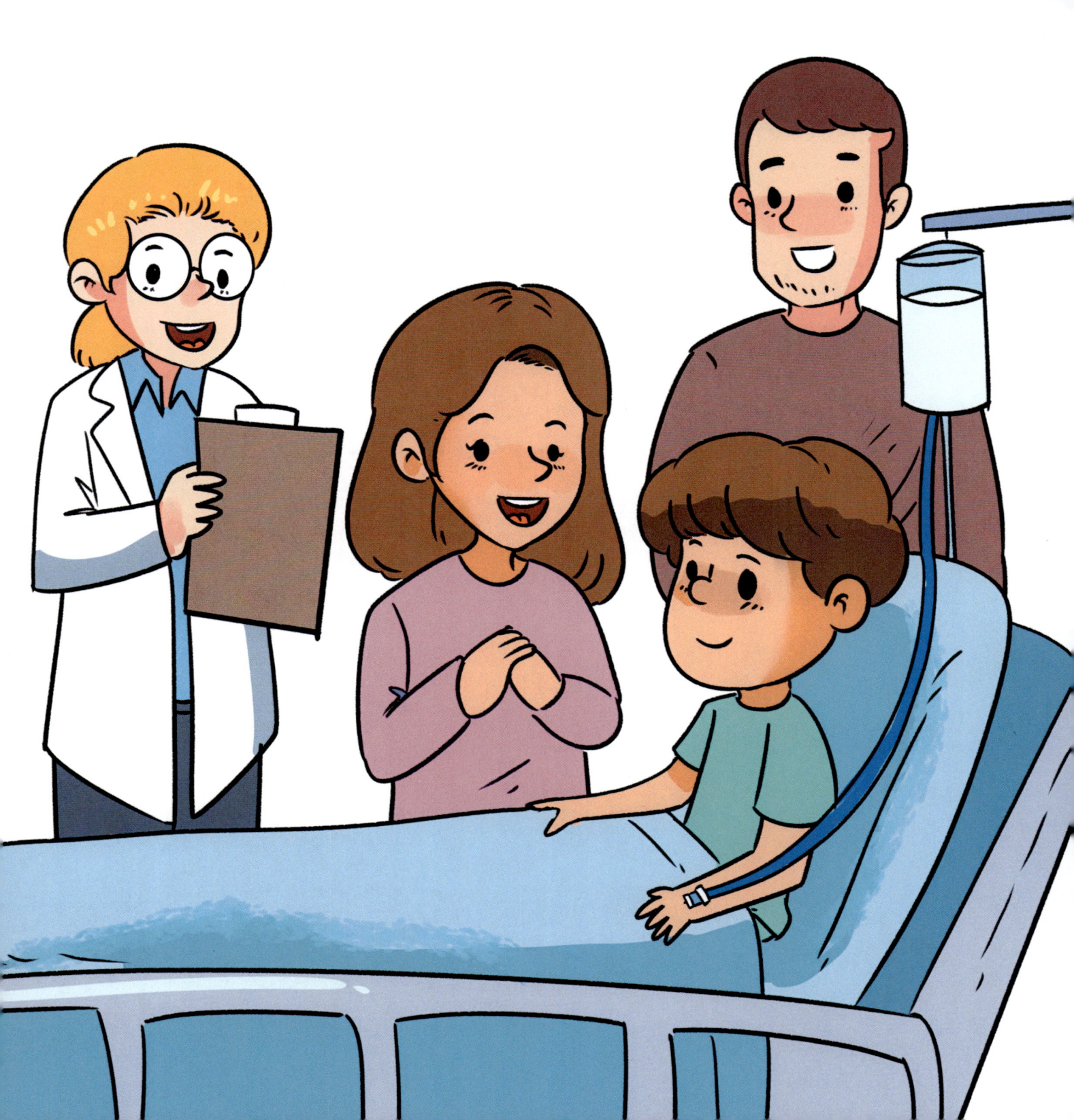

After your adenoids are removed, you will start feeling better soon.

But first, you get to eat ice cream or popsicles, and lots of them, too!

What is your favorite flavor?

_____

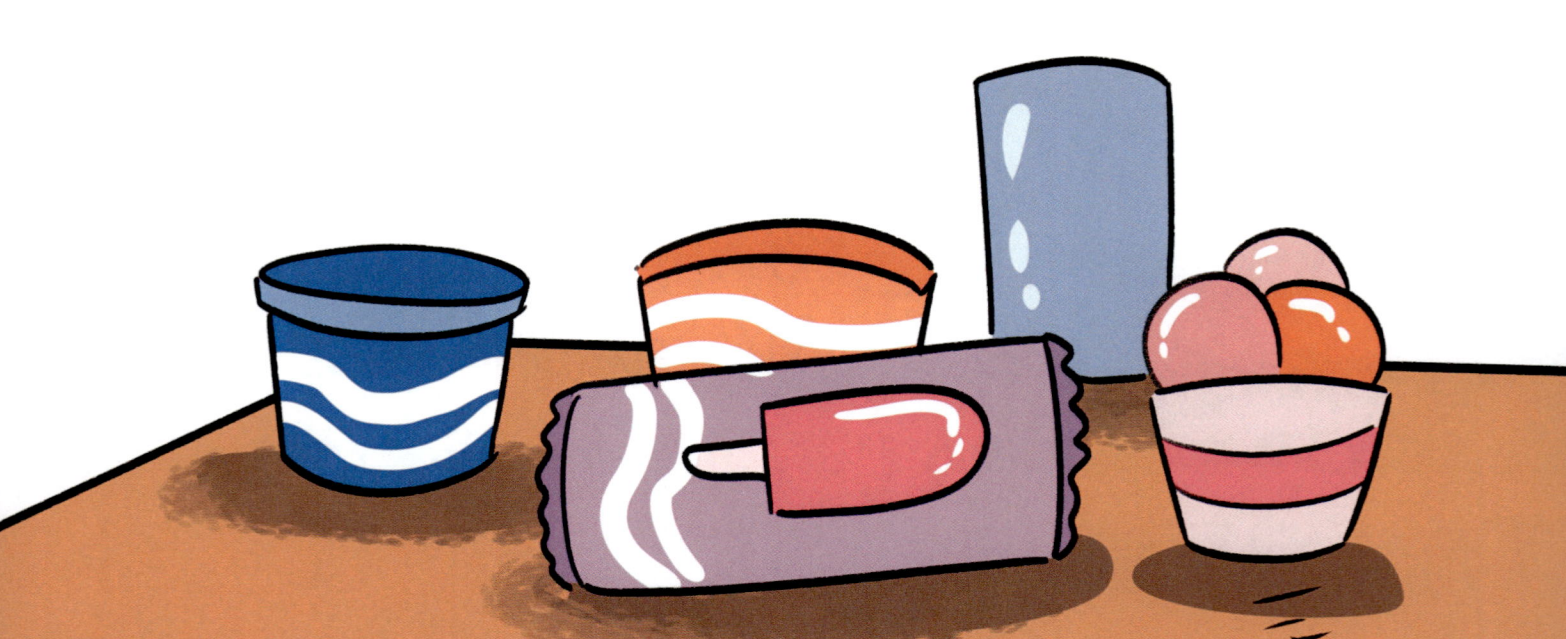

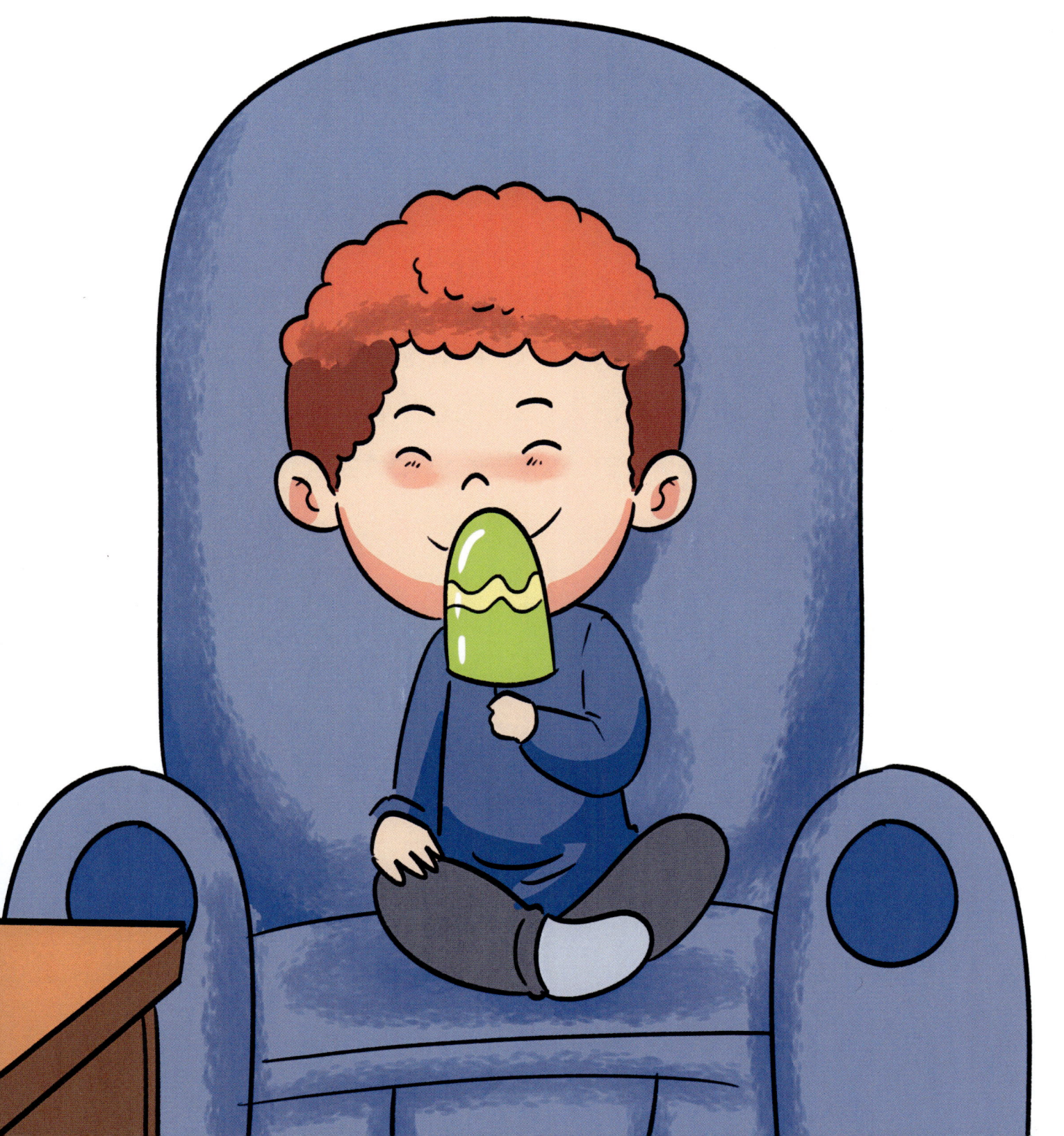

In addition to the ice cream and popsicles, please remember to drink water, juice, or your favorite drink or smoothie to help your body get better sooner.

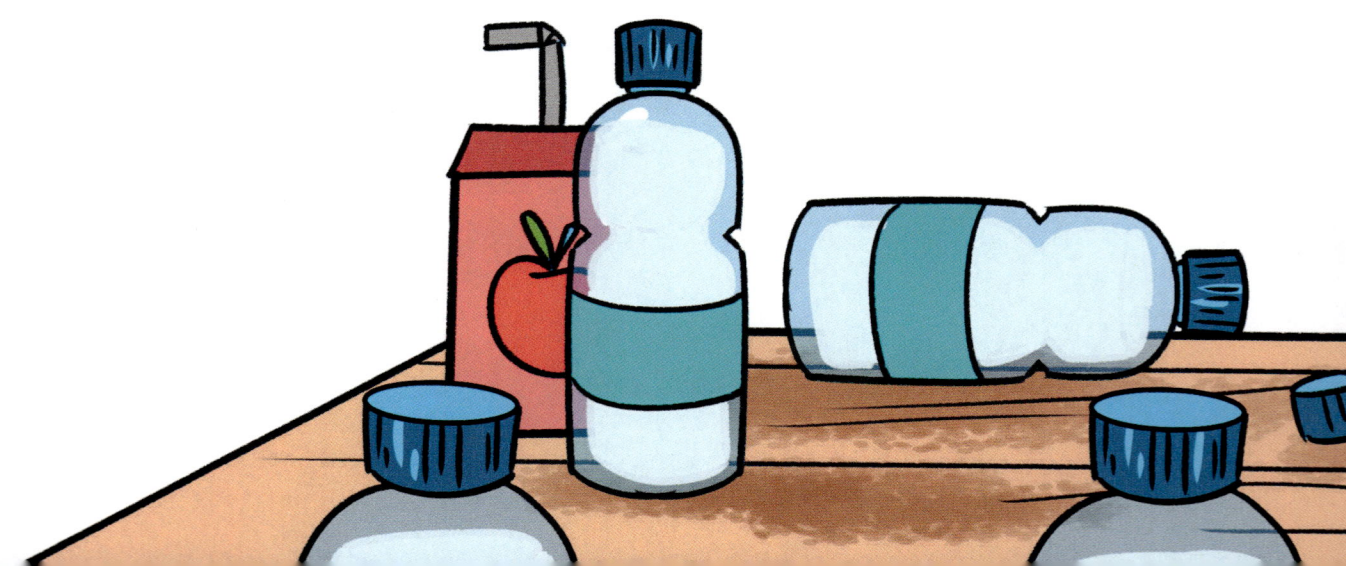

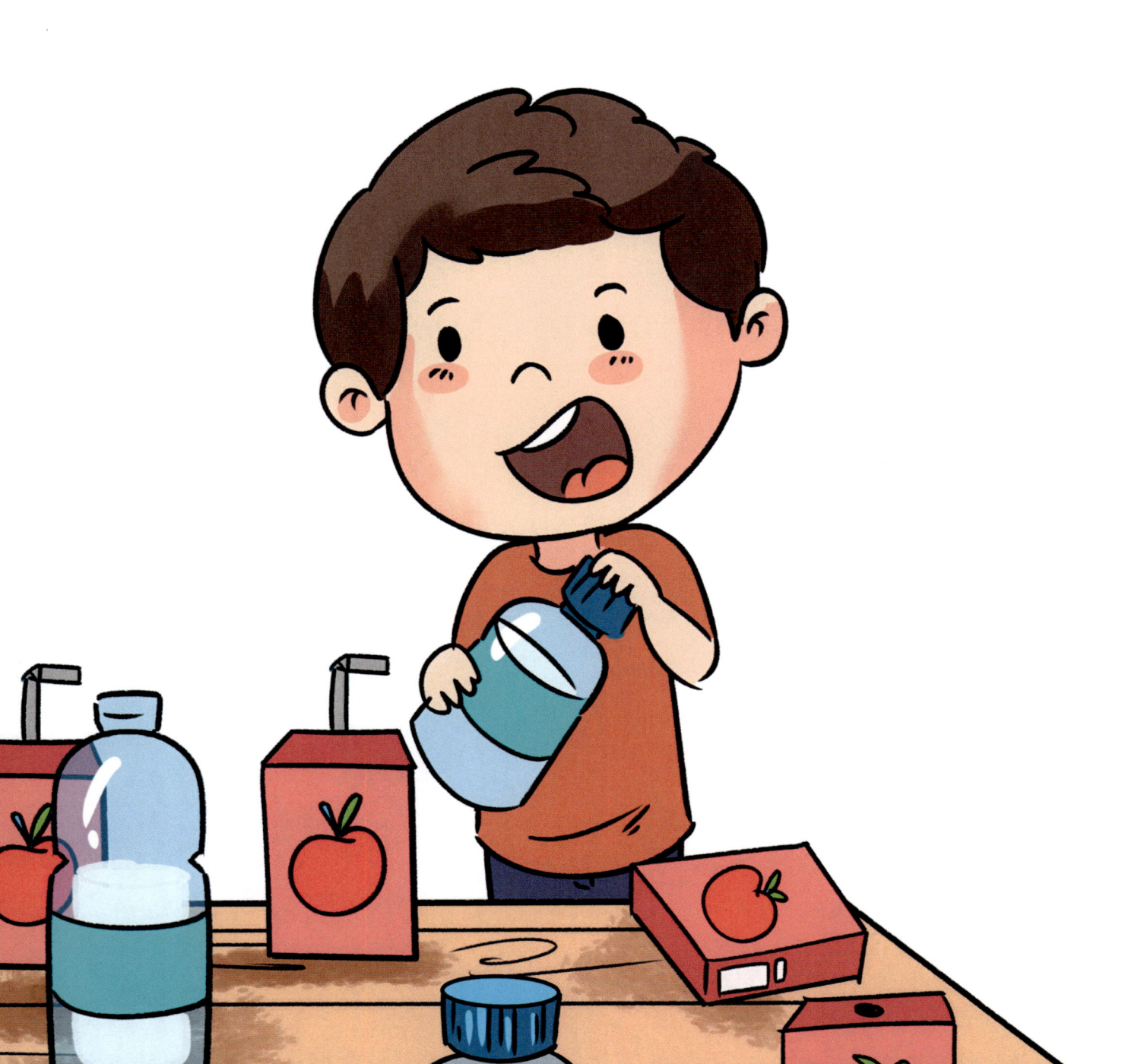

While you're recovering from your surgery, please take it easy.

You can read your favorite books, watch your favorite movies, or play board games.

This is a great time to just *relax* and focus on getting better until you have recovered from your surgery.

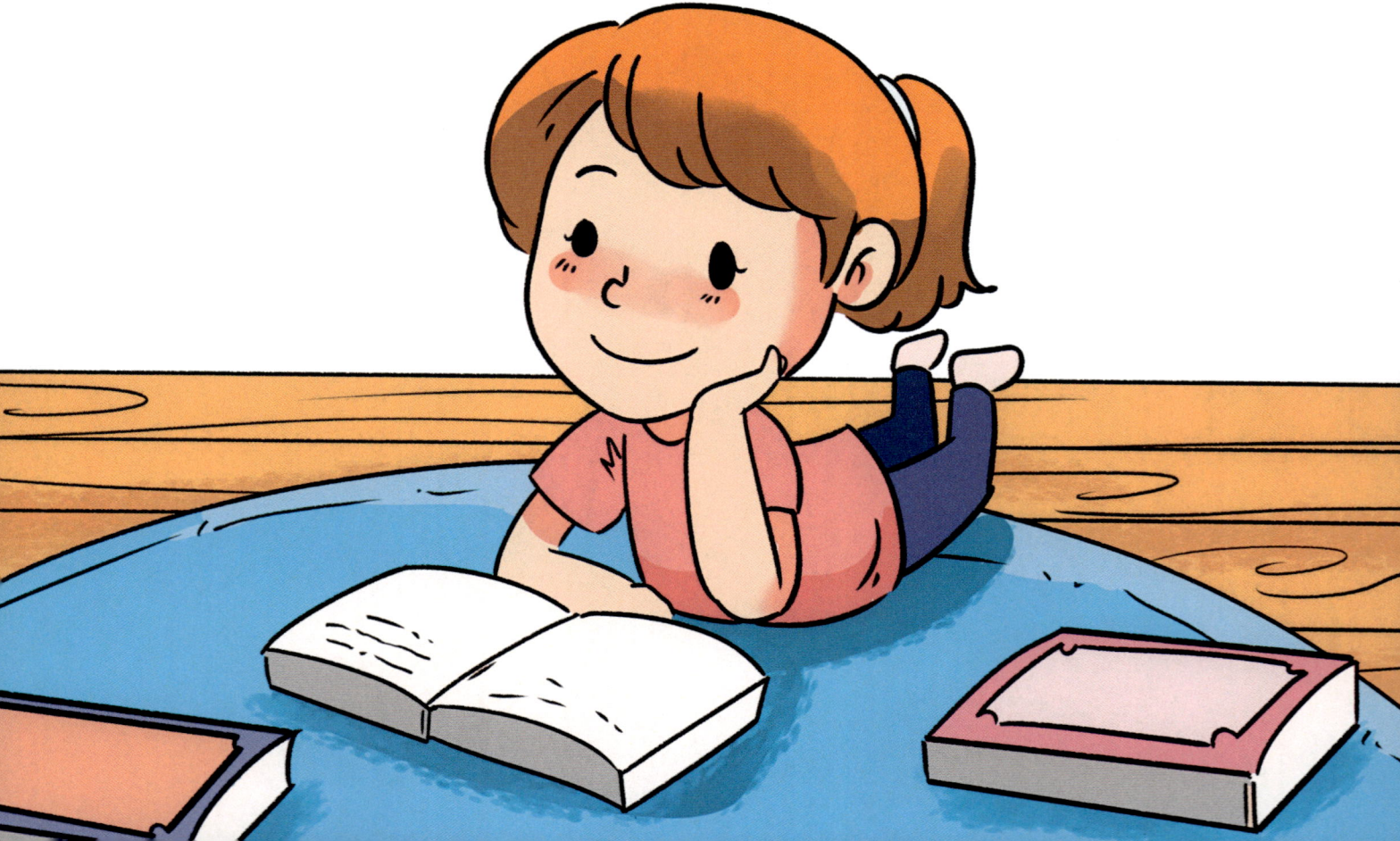

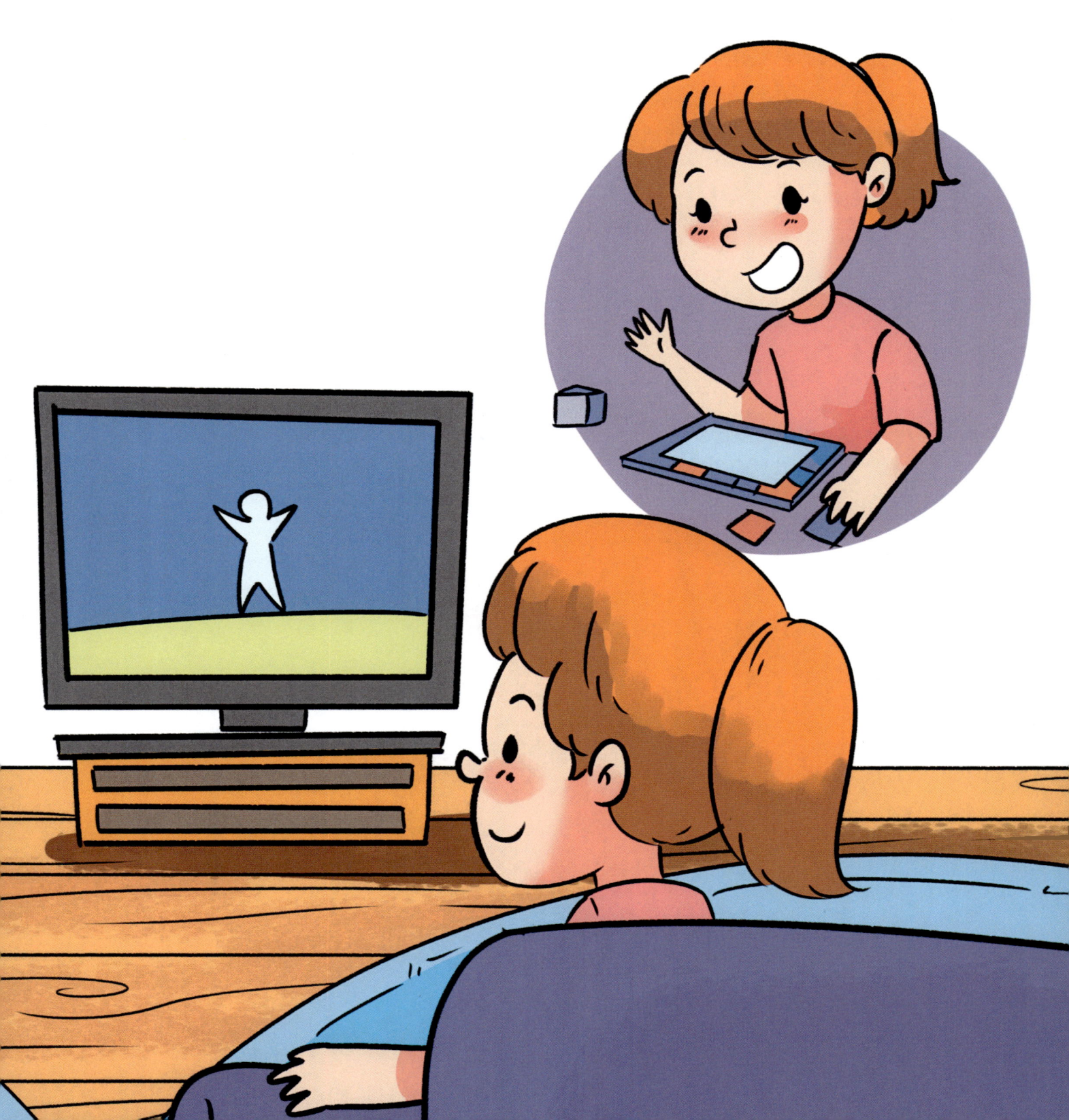

Soon, you will notice you can breathe and feel better, and your throat will not hurt like before.

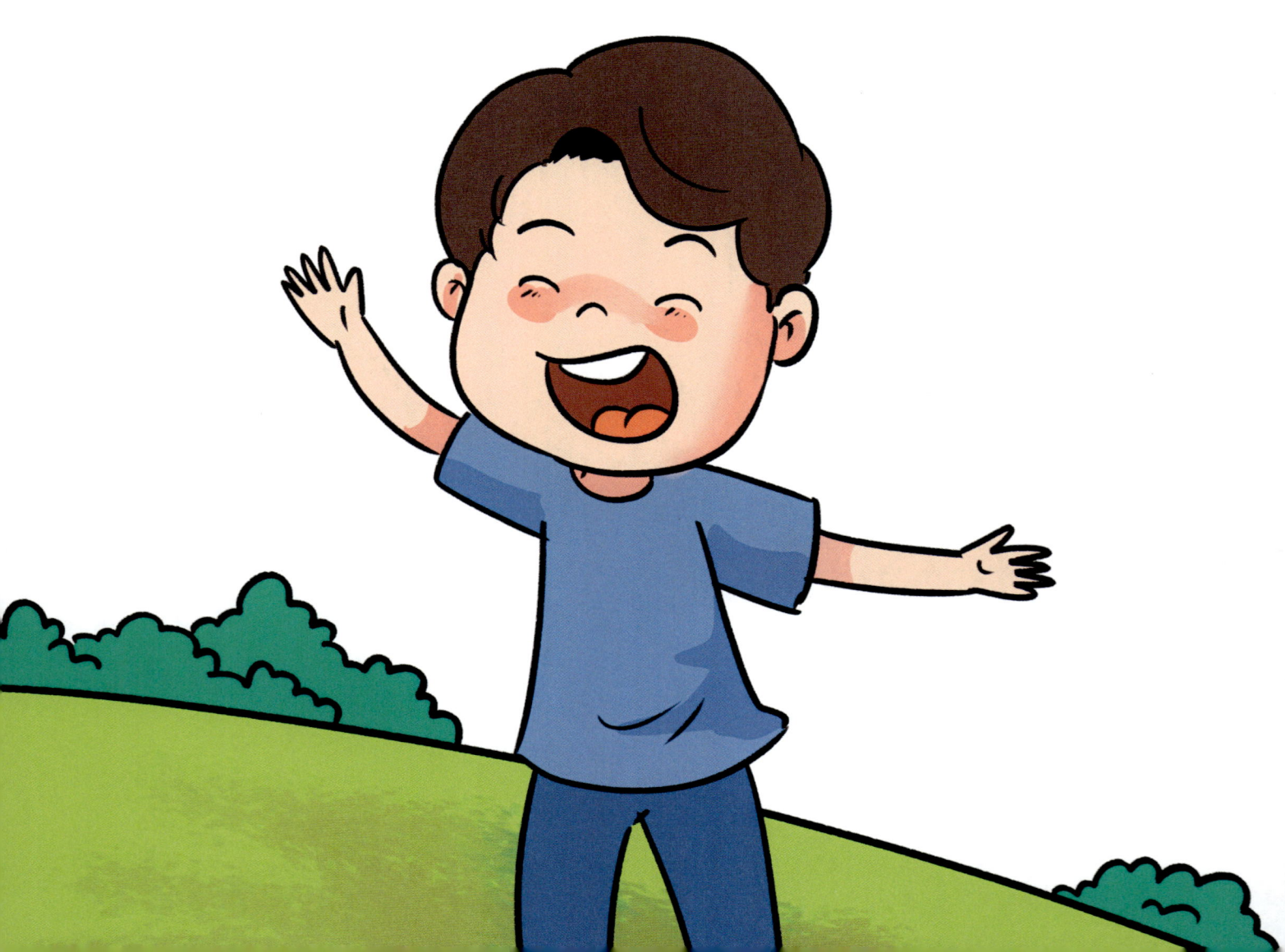

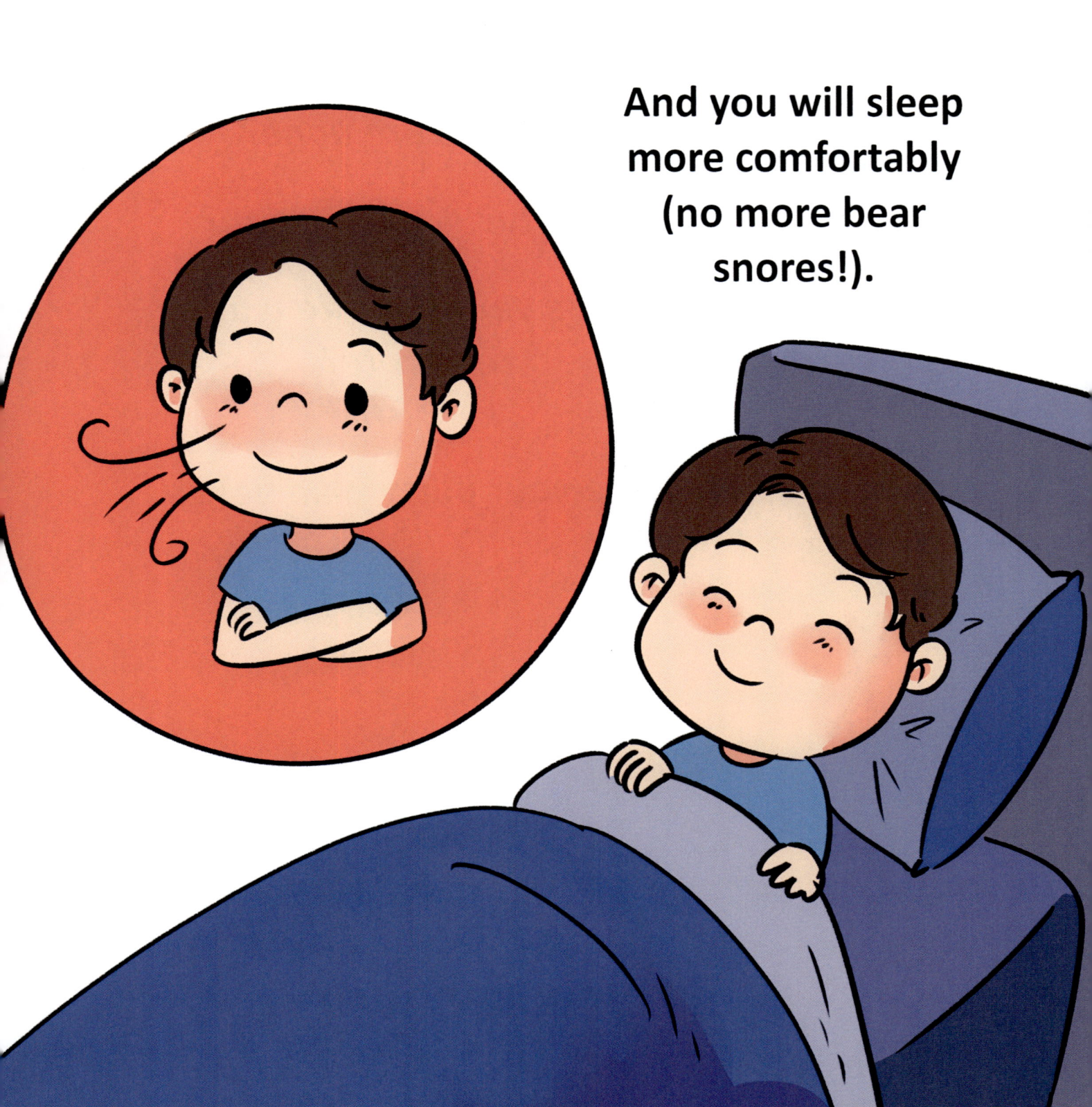

And you will sleep more comfortably (no more bear snores!).

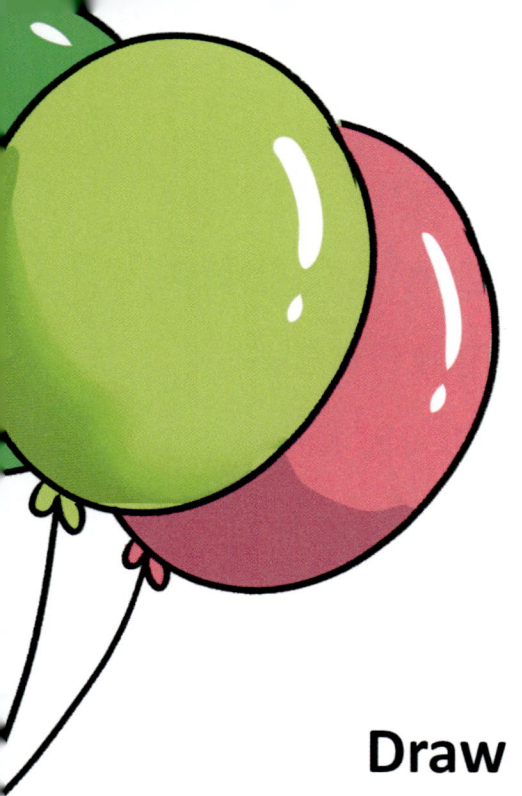

What will you do after your adenoids are gone?

A party? A celebration?

What's your favorite way to celebrate?

Draw or write your party plan below.

Speedy recovery!

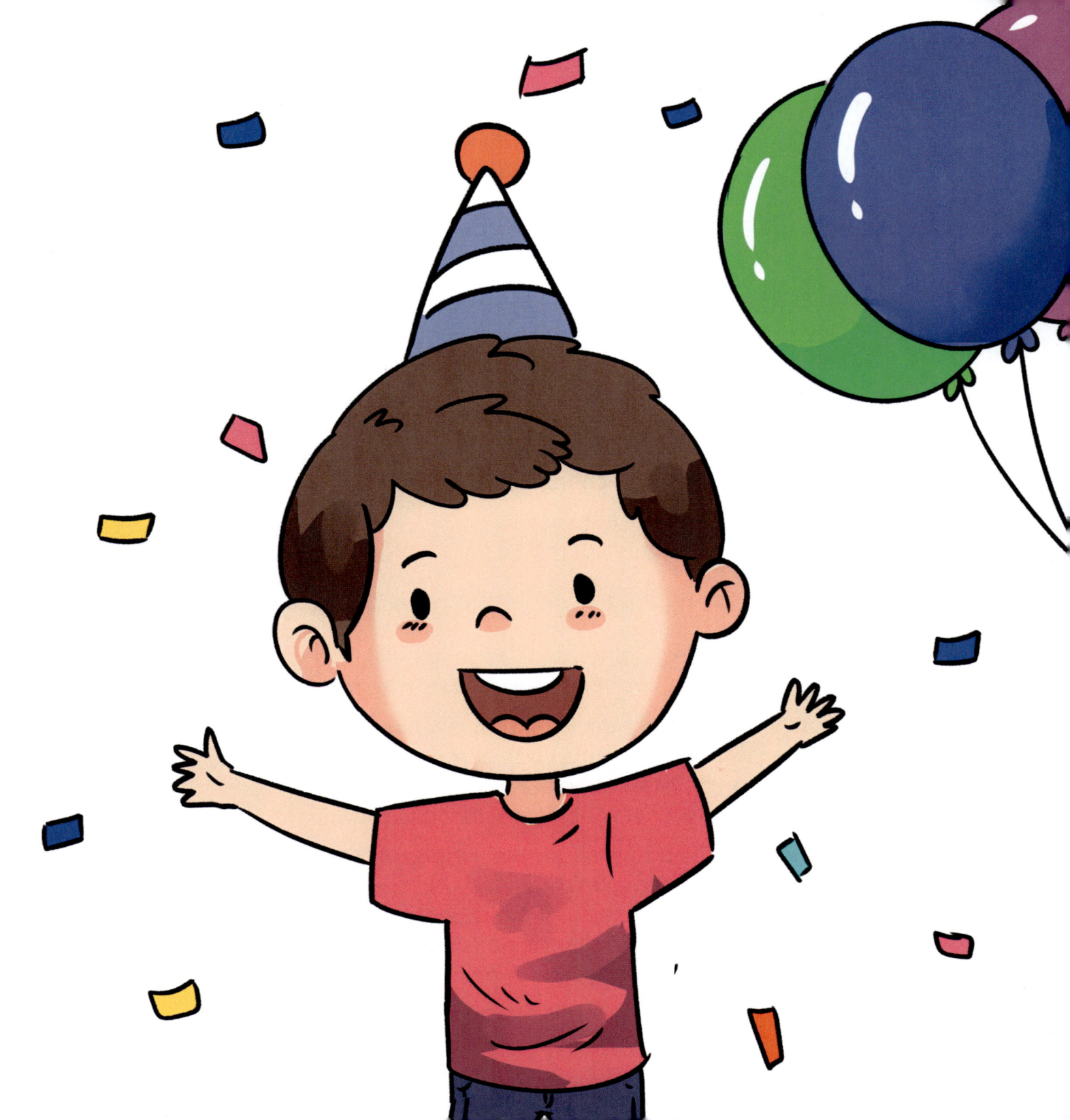

Notes for Parent/Guardian

* Placement of the intravenous (IV) catheter in this young age group is typically done *after* your child is asleep in the operating room.

*After the surgery, it is common for children to feel confused, disoriented, or irritable, and they may cry, sob, kick, scream, or thrash around. It normally takes about one hour for the anesthesia to wear off.

*Post-surgery instructions/restrictions:
Your child's doctor should give you specific instructions on (1) what your child can and cannot do during the recovery period, (2) the duration of the post-surgical restrictions, and (3) any post-surgical follow-ups. Additionally, (4) they should instruct what to watch out for and when it is necessary for you to bring your child back to the hospital in case of an emergency. If they forget, please kindly remind them and obtain these instructions/restrictions before leaving the hospital.

Disclaimer

Please note that the illustrations are not drawn to scale.

This book is written for informational, educational, and personal growth purposes and should not be used as a substitute for medical advice.

Please consult your child's doctor if they need medical attention and to ensure the information in this book pertains to your child's medical condition and needs. I cannot guarantee what your child experiences is exactly what is being discussed in this book.

The author and the publisher are not responsible, either directly or indirectly, for any damages, monetary loss, or reparation due to information in this book. By reading this book, the readers agree not to hold the author and the publisher responsible for any losses as a result of any errors, inaccuracies, or omissions in this book.

Please keep in mind that your child's experience depends on the location, the facility, their medical condition, and the healthcare team. Please use this book in conjunction with your child's doctor's advice. Thank you.

Did this picture book help your child in some way?
If so, I would love to hear about it!

www.amazon.com/gp/product-review/B0DBVCXY5V

For other book titles, please visit:

www.fzwbooks.com

Connect with the author

email: books@fzwbooks.com
facebook/instagram: @FZWbooks

About the Author

Dr. Fei Zheng-Ward is a clinical anesthesiologist who understands the apprehension patients (both adults and children) may have surrounding their upcoming surgery. Her goal in her medical books is to bring useful information to patients so they have a better understanding and appreciation of what happens leading up to, during, and after surgery. She wants readers to be more empowered to make informed decisions and to feel more at ease with their surgery.

As a practicing physician, she takes pride in being respected for her attention to detail, commitment to providing compassionate and personalized patient care, and strong presence in patient advocacy in the perioperative period for each of her patients. She understands the importance of physical and emotional well-being and advocates for patient autonomy.

In addition to her clinical practice, Dr. Zheng-Ward is actively involved in medical education and contributes to medical journals and state and national conferences.

She is an award-winning author for her book titled **What to Expect and How to Prepare for Your Surgery**.

More about Dr. Fei Zheng-Ward:

* Board Certified Anesthesiologist

* Anesthesiology Residency Training at The Johns Hopkins Hospital in Baltimore, MD

* Master in Public Health (MPH) degree from Dartmouth Medical School in Hanover, NH

Books by the author

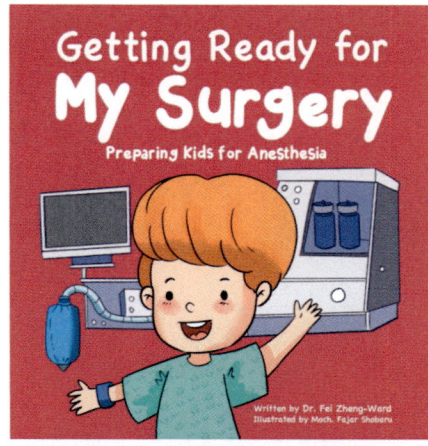
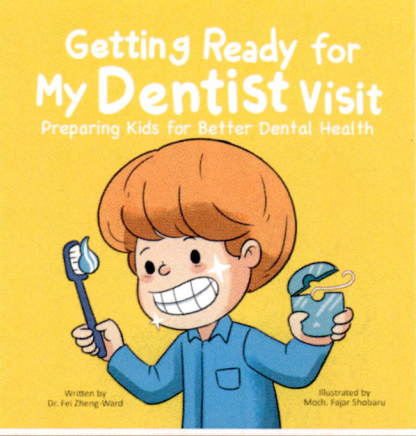
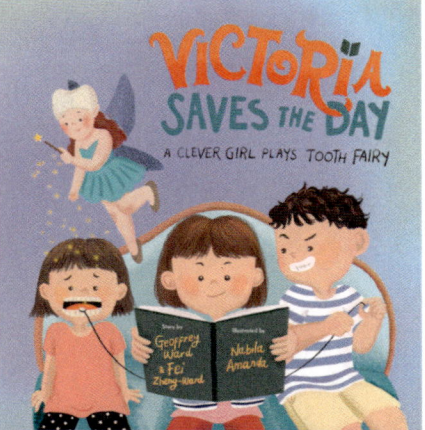
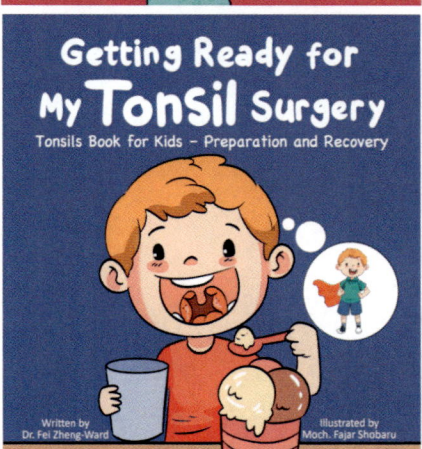
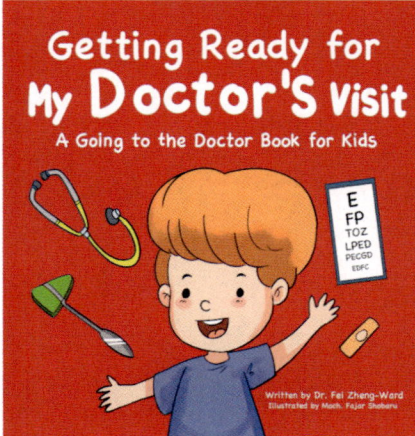
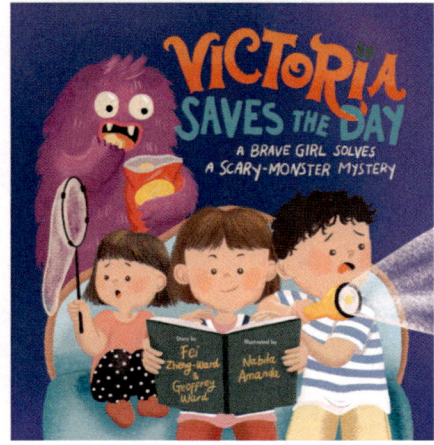
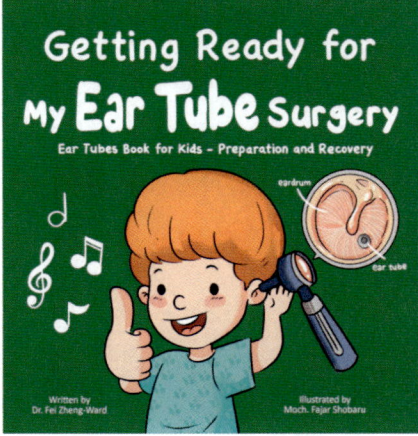
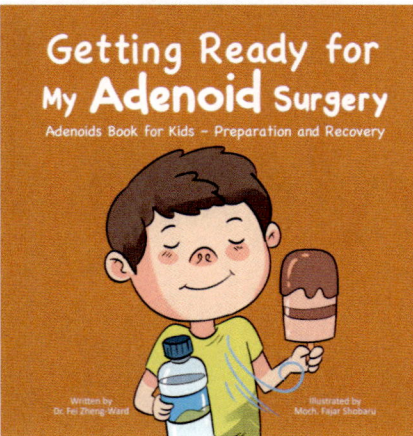
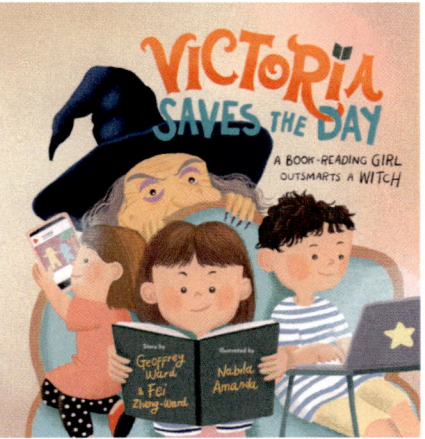

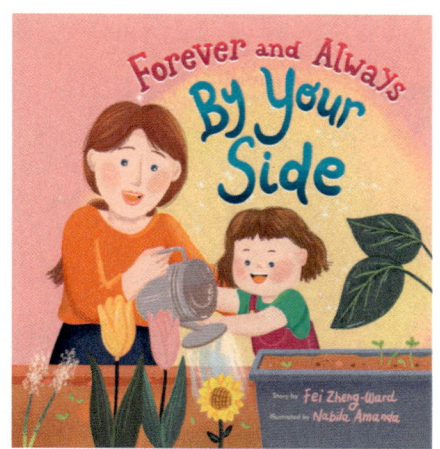
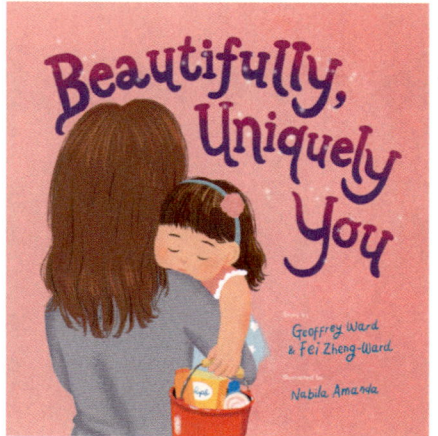
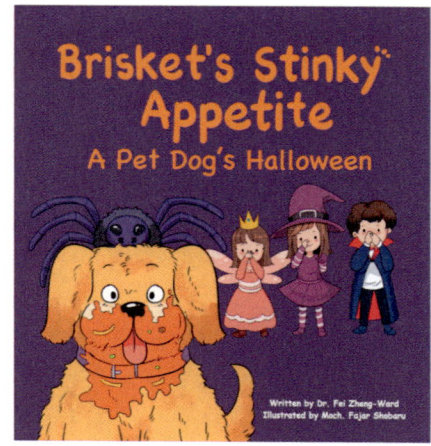
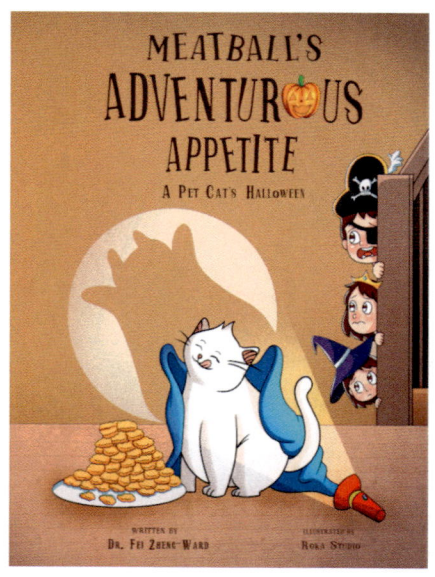
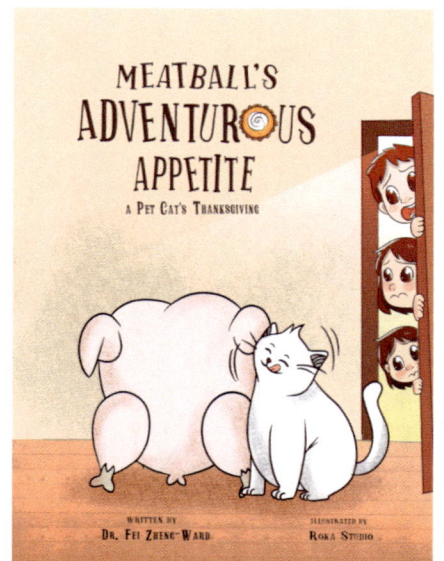
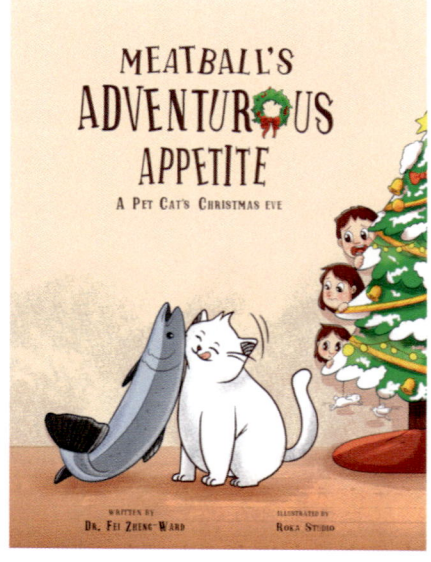
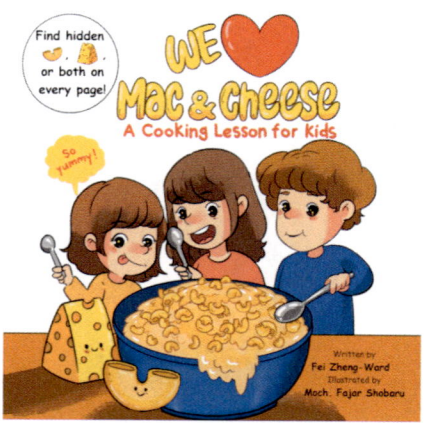
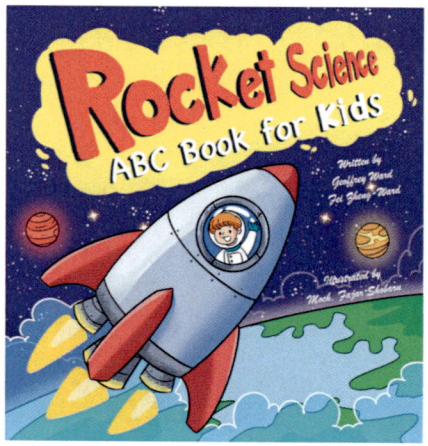
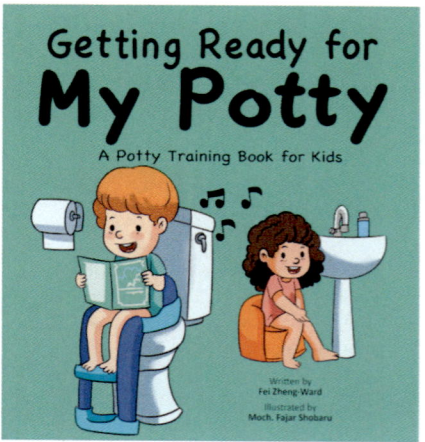

Made in the USA
Las Vegas, NV
07 April 2025